The Functional

MW00443092

The Functional Foot Orthosis

J. W. Philps

RPod(NZ) SRCh(UK) MNZSPod
Course Supervisor, School of Health Sciences (Podiatry),
Central Institute of Technology, Heretaunga, New Zealand

Churchill Livingstone
EDINBURGH LONDON MELBOURNE AND NEW YORK 1990

CHURCHILL LIVINGSTONE
Medical Division of Longman Group UK Limited

Distributed in the United States of America by
Churchill Livingstone Inc., 1560 Broadway, New York,
N.Y. 10036, and by associated companies, branches and
representatives throughout the world.

© J. W. Philps 1990
except Plates 2–9 © Enda McBride 1990

All rights reserved. No part of this publication may be
reproduced, stored in a retrieval system, or transmitted
in any form or by any means, electronic, mechanical,
photocopying, recording or otherwise, without either
the prior written permission of the publishers (Churchill
Livingstone, Robert Stevenson House, 1–3 Baxter's
Place, Leith Walk, Edinburgh EHl 3AF), or a licence
permitting restricted copying in the United Kingdom
issued by the Copyright Licensing Agency Ltd, 33–34
Alfred Place, London, WC1E 7DP.

First published 1990

ISBN 0-443-04058-3

British Library Cataloguing in Publication Data
Philps, J. W.
    The functional foot orthosis.
    1. Medicine. Orthotics
    I. Title
    617'.307

Library of Congress Cataloging in Publication Data
Philps, J. W.
    The functional foot orthosis/J. W. Philps.
        p.   cm.
    Bibliography: p.
    Includes index.
    ISBN 0-443-04058-3
    1. Foot—Abnormalities—Treatment. 2. Orthopedic
    apparatus.
    I. Title.
    [DNLM: 1. Foot. 2. Orthotic Devices. WE 26 P571f]
    RD756.42.P45   1989
    617.5'85—dc20
    DNLM/DLC
    for Library of Congress

Produced by Longman Singapore Publishers (Pte) Ltd
Printed in Singapore

Preface

The functional foot orthosis is a device placed inside a shoe and worn underneath the foot. It is used to synchronise the mechanics of the lower limb by holding the foot in as near to its optimal functioning position as possible. Ideally, at mid-stance, the sub-talar joint is in its neutral position, parallel to the weight-supporting surface. However, it is not always possible to achieve this ideal, particularly in cases where a limited range of motion restricts the movement available between articular surfaces. In these situations a compromise is sought. The functional foot orthosis is an adjunct to many other therapies, including medical, surgical and biomechanical. It can be used in the treatment of foot problems and mechanical problems of the lower limb associated with structural and/or functional abnormalities. It is a concept based on exacting clinical measurement and diagnosis which has been forged from a continuing urge to discover and understand the intricate workings of the human foot, in all its variations. This has led to some headway being made, particularly by podiatrists, in the relief of pain in, and the symptoms associated with, many mechanical faults of the foot and leg.

The functional device can be used for patients of all ages once a clear picture has been developed of an individual's functional ability and limitations. This is achieved by thorough podiatric/orthopaedic examination, encompassing all positional relationships and joint mobility. This examination must be undertaken, for a functional foot orthosis incorrectly prescribed may cause serious damage to the foot of the wearer. Therefore, a clear understanding of the mechanics of the lower limb is paramount, and the text assumes this knowledge in its reader. This book explains the important points involved in the prescription, manufacture and dispensing of the functional foot orthosis. It is intended that the chapters be studied in sequential order, for they are presented in what is, I feel, a logical sequence of development. If followed in this way, the skills gained from each chapter should allow the subsequent material to be understood with ease.

With a sound start, the inevitable practice that will ensue should enable the construction of a device that will meet the therapeutic re-

quirements of the patient and the technical excellence that your professional pride demands.

Heretaunga 1989   J. W. P.

Acknowledgements

I am indebted to my wife, Joanna, for her support and care, and for completing the onerous task of typing the many drafts which invariably result from a project such as this. I am very grateful to our children, Adam, Katy and Thomas, for their understanding and for the time they have been prepared to sacrifice with a father who was often preoccupied.

To two others especially, I owe sincere thanks for the personal time they devoted to this text: Kathy Ansin RPod, MNZSPod, a family friend and podiatrist, whose enviable skills as a practitioner she shared during the many hours spent checking the material for accuracy and clarity; my father, Richard Philps MBE, MD, FRCPath, for his advice, his painstaking examination of the manuscript at all its stages of development, and for the photographs of orthoses contained herein.

It is not possible to thank all those who have given time, counsel and support; these have been many, all of whom will know that my gratitude is sincere. No text would materialise without such friendship.

J. W. Philps

To Joanna

Contents

Introduction

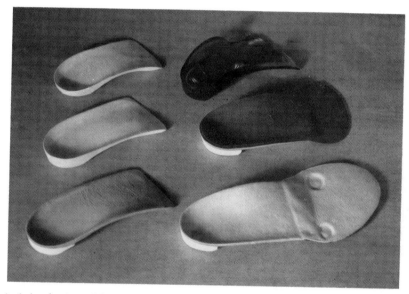

Plate 1 A selection of functional foot orthoses.

Structurally, the functional foot orthosis can be divided into four units.

1. *The shell*

This is usually made of a thermoplastic material which is moulded to a plaster of Paris cast of the plantar surface of the foot (the positive cast of the foot). It is well likened to the frame of a pair of spectacles. The shell, like the spectacle frame, supports the means of correction.

2. *The post*—or correcting platform

This is the material which holds the shell in the functional position desired by the clinician. This may then be likened to the lens of a pair of spectacles because of its corrective function.

3. *The fore-foot extension*

This can also be called an accommodative extension. It consists of a piece of cushioning, or redistributive material, which spans the width and length of the fore-foot, distal to the anterior border of the shell. It is used to improve function and/or redistribute pressure in this area of the plantar surface of the foot.

4. *The cover*

The cover is the final interface placed between the shell of the orthosis and the foot.

There are many materials which are suitable for covering functional foot orthoses; they not only provide aesthetic appeal, but can be used to improve the therapeutic value of the device.

1

Clinical measurements

Any medical treatment aimed at the improvement of a condition, however severe or minor, will only be effective if the patient is examined carefully. If this is done correctly, and the clinician possesses the necessary knowledge, then the resulting diagnosis can be relied upon. This is an essential premise if suitable treatment is to be instigated. It is as critical when considering the use of functional foot orthoses as any other form of treatment. A *complete* biomechanical assessment of the patient is necessary and should never be short-circuited. It should include all the torsional and positional measurements along with the ranges of motion of all the joints of the leg, from the hip downwards. The measurements should be recorded and the decisions made on all aspects of the orthoses while the *patient is still present*. This enables the clinician to check any point that is unclear as the results are evaluated.

It is useful, for peace of mind, as well as being in the interests of continuity and therefore accuracy, if standardisation of the examination and orthosis prescription techniques is achieved. Personally, I record my clinical examination on a specific form of which I then make a precis and transfer to an orthotic prescription form (Fig. 1.1). I have developed this for use at the New Zealand School of Podiatry as a method of double-checking the information required to manufacture the device.

By completing this form a clear picture will be developed of the functional ability of the patient's foot and lower limb. From this, a confident decision can be made on the degree of compensation, correction or torsional adjustment that is required.

HOW THIS DECISION IS MADE

The decision is a complex one, but may be made easier by dividing the limb into four segments:

1. The upper leg (femur)

Student.. Cast satisfactory................. Date Cast taken..................

Patient.......................... No......... Sex.......... Weight..........kg Occupation/Activity....................

Expected Issue Date (to be completed when cast taken).......................Patient's Phone No....................

LOWER LIMB HISTORY	DIAGNOSIS	GENERAL MEDICAL HISTORY AND/OR ANOMALIES
Symptoms .... Lesions Present L....................................... .... R.......................................	L .... R	....

TORSIONAL MEASUREMENTS

Malleolar	L	R
Femoral	L	R

GAIT L [   ] R

Straight	Abducted	Adducted

If excessive Note Angle

L   R

RANGE OF MOTION

	SUB TALAR L R	MID TARSAL L L	FIRST RAY L R	FIRST MPJ L R	ANKLE L R	KNEE L R	HIP L R	STATE DIRECTION
NORMAL	☐ ☐	☐ ☐	☐ ☐	☐ ☐	☐ ☐	☐ ☐	☑ ☑	Internal ☑
EXCESSIVE	☐ ☐	☐ ☐	☐ ☐	☐ ☐	☐ ☐	☐ ☐	☑ ☑	External
LIMITED	☐ ☐	☐ ☐	☑ ☑	☐ ☐	☐ ☐	☐ ☐	☑ ☑	
NONE	☐ ☐	☐ ☐	☐ ☐	☐ ☐	☐ ☐	☐ ☐	☑ ☑	

FIRST RAY NEUTRAL POSITION [L/R]

IF FIRST RAY MOTION IS LIMITED, IN WHICH DIRECTION IS MOVEMENT PRESENT?

DORSIFLEXED [/]   PLANTAR FLEXED [/]   NORMAL [   ]

Dorsiflexion [/]   Plantar flexion

FRONTAL PLANE MEASUREMENTS

	SUB TALAR L R	MID TARSAL L R	TIBIAL STANCE L R	RELAXED CALCANEAL STANCE L R
°VARUS	☐ ☐	☐ ☐	☐ ☐	☐ ☐
°VALGUS	☐ ☐	☐ ☐	☐ ☐	☐ ☐

FRONTAL PLANE MEASUREMENTS (LIMB TO GROUND)

	L	R
REAR FOOT	____ °VARUS ____	
	____ °VALGUS ____	
FORE FOOT	____ °VARUS ____	
	____ °VALGUS ____	

CAST MODIFICATION REQUIRED   **INTRINSIC POSTING** — YES   NO

FIRST RAY ADAPTATIONS

L....................................
....
R....................................
....

ARCHES-WEIGHT-BEARING
LOW MED HIGH
L ☑ ☑ ☑
R ☑ ☑ ☑

ENLARGEMENT OF LESIONS
L....................................
R....................................

IS NORMAL SUB TALAR PRONATION ALLOWED FOR IN ABOVE FORE-FOOT MEASUREMENTS?

YES ☐   NO ☐

ORTHOSES

Shell Material (Tick)
ROHADUR	☐
SUBORTHOLEN	☐
POLYPROPYLENE	☐
EVA	☐
OTHER	

Posting Material
Rear Foot L R   Fore Foot L R
EVA 360	☐ ☐	☐ ☐
EVA 260	☐ ☐	☐ ☐
EVA 220	☐ ☐	☐ ☐
ACRYLIC	☐ ☐	☐ ☐
OTHER............		

Top Cover
NONE	☐
TO WEBBING	☐
FULL LENGTH	☐

Cover Material
LEATHER	☐
VINYL	☐
FOAM VINYL	☐
3mm STARLITE	☐
3mm STARPRENE	☐
OTHER	

Accomodative Extension

NOTES
....
....
....

FITTING Dated...................

Signed...........................

WEAR CHECK Signed...........................

Date.................... Points to note...........................

Fig. 1.1 Podiatry Functional Orthosis Prescription Form

2. The lower leg (tibia and fibula)
3. The rear-foot (structures proximal to the mid-tarsal joint)
4. The fore-foot (structures distal to the mid-tarsal joint).

The posting angulation is based on the relationships of these segments upon one another, and their combined relationship with the supporting surface. The relationships are as follows:

a. The frontal and transverse plane relationships of the upper leg to the lower leg

b. The frontal and transverse plane relationships of the lower leg to the ground

c. The frontal, transverse and sagittal plane relationships of the rear-foot to the lower leg

d. The frontal, transverse and sagittal plane relationships of the fore-foot to the rear-foot.

Remember this statement:

The posting angulation is based on the relationships of these segments upon one another, and their *combined relationship with the supporting surface.*

The path through this maze of decisions is made more clear by grasping this one initial concept, i.e. that the limb is functioning on the ground. Therefore, whatever measurements result from the examination, the measurement that is of ultimate concern is *the angle, in the frontal plane, that the foot makes with the ground at mid-stance with the sub-talar joint in its neutral position.* It is assumed, for the purpose of the examination, that the ground is level. The measurements that give this reading are above all else:

1. The tibial stance measurement
2. The sub-talar joint measurment
3. The mid-tarsal joint measurement.

However, these readings cannot be isolated from one another, or directly from:

a. The torsional measurements of the whole limb. These alter the transverse plane relationship of the foot to the ground.
b. The ranges of motion of all the joints associated with gait, including the hip joint. These alter the limb's ability to move in any one direction and its ability to compensate for an abnormal positional relationship.
   A full awareness of the normal ranges of motion of the joints involved is, of course, fundamental.
c. Muscle imbalance which may change positional relationships during function.

Any one of (a), (b) or (c) may increase or decrease the frontal plane angular relationship of the foot with the ground. Consequently, they are as vital as any other measurement.

TRANSLATION OF CLINICAL MEASUREMENTS INTO POSTING ANGLES

To achieve the necessary angulation of an orthosis requires an ability to perform a detailed biomechanical assessment of the lower limb and then to translate the functional ability and angular measurements taken during the examination into posting angles.

Of fundamental importance in the translation is the ability to interpret the measurements which indicate the frontal plane angulation of the foot with the ground. As mentioned already, these are: the tibial stance, the sub-talar and mid-tarsal joint measurements (angles). Each of these angles registers the position of the individual segments which combine geometrically to decide the angle at which the foot should function on the ground at mid-stance, e.g. if the sub-talar joint is in its neutral position and there is no abnormality in the angulation of the calcaneus (the sub-talar angle), or the fore-foot (the mid-tarsal joint angle) and the tibia is perpendicular to the ground, the plantar surface of the foot will be parallel to the ground. However, if the sub-talar and mid-tarsal joint angles remain unchanged with respect to the leg, but the tibia is angled by 6 degrees in the frontal plane, then the foot will also be angled by the same amount if the sub-talar joint is to maintain its neutral position. The interrelationship is shown in Figure 1.2.

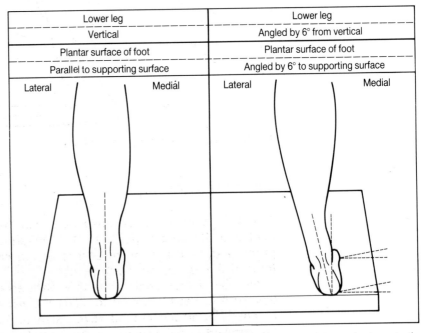

Lower leg	Lower leg
Vertical	Angled by 6° from vertical
Plantar surface of foot	Plantar surface of foot
Parallel to supporting surface	Angled by 6° to supporting surface
Lateral Medial	Lateral Medial

Fig. 1.2. Left leg viewed from behind. The angulation of the tibia results in a similar angulation of the foot if the sub-talar joint is to maintain its neutral position.

If one accepts this concept, then it follows that the frontal plane relationship and degree of angulation of each individual segment has, because of the articulations between each one of them, the potential to affect the other two and overall, the angle at which the foot functions with the ground.

Therapeutically the aim is to develop the optimal combined angulation of the three segments so that when they are combined, the most *efficient* functional position of the limb is achieved. (This may not always be the most 'normal'.)

When translation of clinical measurements is first undertaken, the process will become more logical if some thought is given to the method by which the angles were measured. By examining and calculating the three measurements mentioned, their relationship to one another will be understood and the 'pure' frontal plane posting angles for an orthosis will be achieved.

TIBIAL STANCE (Fig. 1.3)

This is measured from the ground using a tractograph, and is the number of degrees that the tibia deviates from a vertical. It is measured while the patient is standing and the sub-talar joint is in its neutral position.

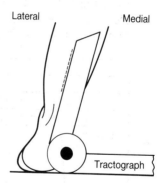

Lateral   Medial

Tractograph

Fig. 1.3 Tibial stance. Left leg viewed from behind.

SUB-TALAR ANGLE (Fig. 1.4)

This is the angle the calcaneus makes with the tibia when the sub-talar joint is in its neutral position. It is measured with the patient lying prone and by using the bisections of the calcaneus and lower one-third of the leg, as reference points.

Because of their anatomical interrelationship, any angulation of the tibia or calcaneus is bound to affect the angle at which the calcaneus functions upon the ground at mid-stance. The effect will depend on the similarity or difference in the frontal plane positions of either of these two segments. Thus if they are similar, they will compound to

Lateral   Medial

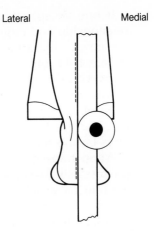

Fig. 1.4 Sub-talar angle. Left leg viewed from above.

enlarge the overall angle; if they are in opposing frontal plane positions, one angle will tend to reduce the other or totally counteract it. For example:

		or
Tibial stance	= 6 degrees varus	6 degrees varus
Sub-talar joint angle	= 3 degrees varus	3 degrees valgus
Overall angulation of rear-foot when measured from a vertical with the ground	= 9 degrees varus	3 degrees varus

REAR-FOOT ANGLE

This is the calculation of the tibial stance and sub-talar joint measurements. The angle is calculated from a vertical and is the 'pure' angle to which the rear-foot can be posted (see Fig. 1.8).

MID-TARSAL JOINT ANGLE (Fig. 1.5)

This is the angle that the fore-foot makes with the bisection line of the calcaneus, with the patient lying prone and the mid-tarsal joint fully 'locked'. The angle is established by noting the number of degrees the fore-foot varies from a line perpendicular to the bisection on the posterior surface of the calcaneus. It is measured using the plantar surface of the metatarsophalangeal joints as the reference line.

FORE-FOOT ANGLE

This is the combined total of the rear-foot angle and the mid-tarsal

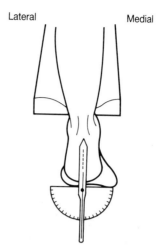

Fig. 1.5 Mid-tarsal joint angle. Left leg viewed from above.

joint angle. It is measured from a horizontal and is the 'pure' angle to which the fore-foot can be posted (see Fig. 1.9).

As has been stressed, alteration in any one of the segments constituting this accumulated angular relationship will affect the angle at which the whole foot is presented to the ground and inevitably its functional efficiency.

The angular relationships and calculations of posting angles can be worked out by simple mathematics. However, it is sometimes easier when first attempting this work, to visualise these relationships by drawing a linear diagram of the leg in the frontal plane. It is easiest to visualise the leg, viewed as it was examined, from behind. The basic layout of the linear diagram is shown in Figure 1.6.

To complete the diagram accurately you will require a pencil, a ruler and a protractor. It may now be helpful to develop the diagram in stages. (All the subsequent diagrams are of a left leg viewed from behind.)

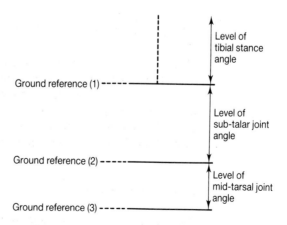

Fig. 1.6

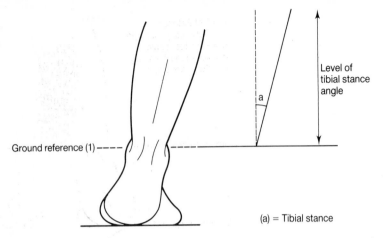

Ground reference (1)

Level of
tibial stance
angle

(a) = Tibial stance

Fig. 1.7

The first thing to draw in is the tibia, angled as it was, from vertical (the tibial stance). (This is measured from a vertical to 'Ground reference' (1) (Fig. 1.7).

Because of the influence the tibial stance will have on the angle at which the rear-foot is placed upon the ground, the line depicting the position of the tibia must be continued (for the sake of the diagram) below the horizontal line of 'Ground reference' (1), from which it was measured. This will produce the reference line from which to measure the sub-talar joint angle. The rear-foot angle is eventually established by measuring the angle from vertical that the line drawn to depict the sub-talar joint angle (the bisection of the calcaneus) makes with 'Ground reference' (2) (Fig. 1.8).

The mid-tarsal joint angle is now inserted on the diagram. This is done by drawing a reference line perpendicular to the line depicting the bisection of the calcaneus which was used to measure the angle

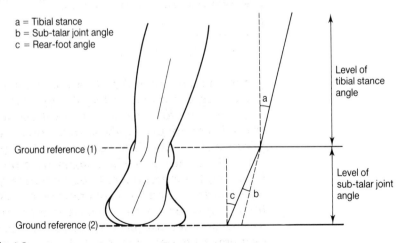

a = Tibial stance
b = Sub-talar joint angle
c = Rear-foot angle

Level of
tibial stance
angle

Ground reference (1)

Level of
sub-talar joint
angle

Ground reference (2)

Fig. 1.8

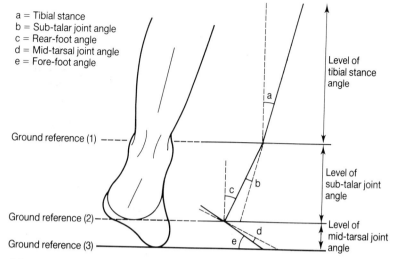

a = Tibial stance
b = Sub-talar joint angle
c = Rear-foot angle
d = Mid-tarsal joint angle
e = Fore-foot angle

Level of tibial stance angle

Ground reference (1)

Level of sub-talar joint angle

Ground reference (2)

Level of mid-tarsal joint angle

Ground reference (3)

Fig. 1.9

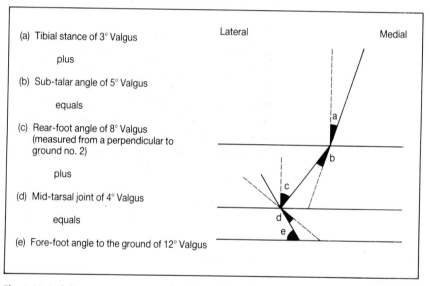

(a) Tibial stance of 3° Valgus

plus

(b) Sub-talar angle of 5° Valgus

equals

(c) Rear-foot angle of 8° Valgus (measured from a perpendicular to ground no. 2)

plus

(d) Mid-tarsal joint of 4° Valgus

equals

(e) Fore-foot angle to the ground of 12° Valgus

Lateral

Medial

Fig. 1.10 Left leg (posterior view).

of the sub-talar joint. A further line is then drawn at the correct number of degrees deviation that the fore-foot makes from the reference line. The fore-foot angle is then established by measuring the angle that this line (depicting the plantar surface of the metatarsophalangeal joints) makes with 'Ground reference' (3) (Fig. 1.9).

For clarity, the preceding angles have been developed sequentially. However, the measurements would normally all be inserted on the one diagram, and I think it would now be of value to study some of these. Initially, measurements which are in the same frontal plane relationship to one another will be used (Figs 1.10 and 1.11—the angles on the diagrams have been exaggerated for clarity).

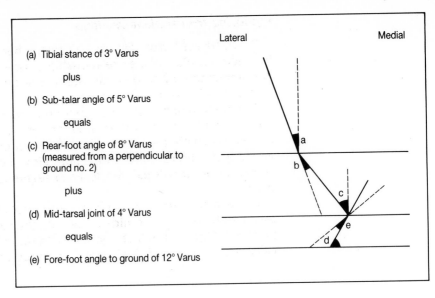

Fig. 1.11 Left leg (posterior view).

Having studied the preceding diagrams, it should be possible to deduce clearly that when the measurements are all in the same frontal plane relationship they accumulate, thus enlarging the angle at which the foot functions with the ground. Therefore, they are added together to give the resulting rear-foot and fore-foot angles. However, this is not so when the measurements differ in their frontal plane relationships, as one reading partially or totally counteracts the other (Fig. 1.12).

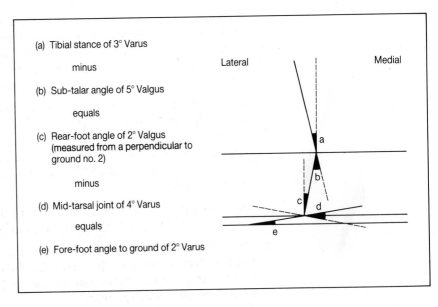

Fig. 1.12 Left leg (posterior view).

Opposing frontal plane readings

It can be seen from Figure 1.12 that, when the measurements differ in their frontal plane relationships, one measurement tends to counteract the other to some extent. Therefore, they are subtracted to give the rear-foot and fore-foot angles.

The method of line drawings explained here is a useful way of visualising the frontal plane angular relationship of the foot as it functions at mid-stance, with the sub-talar joint in its neutral position. When therapy is being considered, these diagrams allow a clear picture to be gained of exactly what will happen to each segment by adjusting any one of them.

The measurements gained from these calculations are the 'pure' angles assumed by the foot at mid-stance with the sub-talar joint in its neutral position. One factor that can affect these calculations is the 'relaxed calcaneal stance' and it will now be discussed.

RELAXED CALCANEAL STANCE

The relaxed calcaneal stance is an indication of the way the foot is compensating for a positional anomaly of one or more segments. In relaxed calcaneal stance the calcaneus will tilt in the direction which the normal range of motion at its articular surfaces allows, in order that the whole weight-bearing surface of the foot can achieve ground contact.

However:

1. Muscle imbalances may prevent this motion from occurring.
2. Excessive varus positional anomalies of either fore- or rear-foot may prevent full ground contact by the foot. The range of motion, particularly at the sub-talar joint, may not be sufficient for this to be achieved, and may create two possible situations:

   a. The fore-foot will adapt to support the anomaly, often by plantar-flexing the first toe or first ray.
   b. The femur and tibia can externally rotate and the knee flex, causing the foot to abduct. This enables the calcaneus to evert *on the ground* to an angle greater than could be achieved by its normal range of motion.

3. Valgus positional anomalies of the limb to the ground, or the fore-foot to the rear-foot, demonstrate three effects in relaxed stance:

   a. The calcaneus can invert, indicating a fixed valgus deformity at the fore-foot relative to the rear-foot. This may be mistaken for a fixed plantar-flexed deformity of the first ray, the possibility of which should be eliminated.
   b. The valgus position of the calcaneus may remain static indicating

that the range of motion at the sub-talar and mid-tarsal joints have been extended to their full limits.

   c. The calcaneal valgus positioning may increase, indicating that a range of motion is still present in some of the joints associated with gait. The joints involved will be seen on examination.

4. Some patients will have a valgus position of one joint opposing a varus position of another. This gives a permutation which can be worked out easily by the method of frontal plane line drawings already shown.

It would be difficult to describe all the variations that may occur in relaxed stance. I have attempted to give a few, so that the thought process is seeded in your mind. The factors initiating the variations are listed at the beginning of this chapter. The resultant relaxed stance, limb to ground measurement in the frontal plane is achieved by the ability the limb has to compensate for an anomaly.

SUMMARY

To establish posting angles it is necessary to *add* similar frontal plane readings and *deduct* dissimilar ones, i.e. varus plus varus and valgus plus valgus **but** varus *minus* valgus.

   The posting angles are needed to establish the angle the foot makes to the ground with the sub-talar joint in its neutral position. To do this one may say:

Tibial stance plus or minus sub-talar joint
measurement   = *Rear-foot angle*

Rear-foot angle plus or minus mid-tarsal
joint measurement   = *Fore-foot angle*

   These angles are indicative of the *correct* mid-stance relationship of the foot to the ground, i.e. they do not indicate the relaxed compensated stance the patient may assume on weight bearing which can, of course, be altered by any one deformity that may be present.

   Posting aims to hold the foot in as near to its correct mid-stance relationship as is possible and thus to allow more normal articular function from this position. However, when the prescription is being written, three further considerations must be borne in mind regarding the posting angles.

1. Excessive frontal plane deformities in the leg can result in the accumulated rear-foot angle becoming too excessive to post realistically. This is because of the inherent restrictions placed upon you technically, by the amount of room available in a conventional shoe which prevents large frontal plane twisting of the foot. Therefore the maximum amount the rear-foot can be posted to is 8 degrees.

2. A limited range of motion at the sub-talar joint, or other joints associated with gait may prevent the proper mid-stance relationship of the foot from being achieved. In these cases the most suitable therapeutic compromise must be sought.

3. Realignment in the elderly person, after many years of poor alignment, cannot sometimes be achieved quickly. In this instance it is prudent to discount the tibial stance measurement initially, when equating the rear-foot posting angulation. Correct alignment must be sought in manageable stages until the therapeutic ideal is reached. Careful manipulation of the weight to thickness ratio of the materials chosen for the orthosis (Ch. 2) may enable more pliable materials to be used to gain the therapeutic advantage desired.

SAGITTAL PLANE ANGULATION OF POSTS

If an unusual sagittal plane angulation of the orthosis is necessary, e.g. because of equinus, the amount of heel raise that is required to enable the heel to bear weight must be noted. This will affect the sagittal plane angulation of the posts (see pp. 79 and 95).

2

Choice of material

In this chapter the basic classification of materials used for the shells and 'posts' of orthoses will be described.

SHELL OF THE ORTHOSIS

The materials used to manufacture the shells of functional foot orthoses fall into three categories:

1. **Rigid**
   Rohadur[1]
2. **Semi-flexible–flexible**
   Subortholen[1]
   Polypropylene[2]
   Acrylonitrile butadiene styrene (ABS)
   Aquaplast[3]
   Sansplint[4]
3. **Cushioning–accommodative**
   Ethylene vinyl acetate (EVA).

'POST' OF THE ORTHOSIS

The properties of the materials used to manufacture the 'posts' of functional foot orthoses also fall into three categories. The properties may be used individually or collectively if a multiple function is required of the post, i.e. shock-absorbing on heel strike but possessing firm pronatory control at mid-stance.

1. **Rigid**
   Dental acrylic
   This can only be used on rigid shell materials otherwise it will shear free from the material.

2. **Semi-rigid**
   High density (360) Ethylene vinyl acetate
   This is used to give rigid and semi-flexible shells, firm rear-foot control. It may be reinforced if necessary by the insertion of nylon screws, epoxy resin, dental acrylic or wooden dowelling on the side of maximum stress.

3. **Shock-absorbing**
   Medium density (220–260) Ethylene vinly acetate.
   This can also have nylon screws, epoxy resin or dental crylic inserted in the side of maximum stress if shock absorbancy and good joint control are the functions required.

The technical details and properties of these materials are dealt with in Chapter 6.

HOW THE CHOICE OF MATERIAL IS MADE

The choice is always governed by the *amount of control required*. The more rigid the material, the more control will be achieved within the joints of the foot.

This choice can be influenced by:

a. The thickness of the material chosen to make the shell
b. The density of the material chosen to control the position of the orthosis in the shoe, the post
c. The weight of the patient.

It is a clinical decision and is based on the assessment, diagnosis and aims of treatment.

'WEIGHT TO THICKNESS RATIO'

The thickness of a material will influence its function. It is accepted that the rigidity of most materials is directly proportional to their thickness and that their flexibility is inversely proportional.

It is not possible to standardise this statement, however, because the qualities a material exhibits under stress must also relate to the forces attempting to distort it.

It can generally be expected that the greater the forces acting on a material, the greater will be the distortion noticed in it. A fine line, technically, is drawn between optimum flexibility for weight and actual fracture or failure of a material. The failure of a material can be due to poor manufacturing techniques, but it is invariably due to the forces tending to distort the material being too great for the thickness of material prescribed.

This concept I term the 'weight to thickness ratio'. It involves a slightly more complex thought pattern than it initially seems, because the actual forces involved in kinesiology have to be considered before a decision is made. The forces to which the orthosis is subjected are the potential forces of body weight combined with the kinetic forces of movement. These kinetic forces increase the potential force many times.

The 'weight to thickness ratio' must be considered when relating the patient's weight and activity, together with the aims of treatment, to the materials available.

The thicknesses of the materials mentioned in Table 2.1 relate the patient's weight to the qualities the materials will exhibit under stress. Many permutations may be created from this table as will be explained later.

Table 2.1   Shell materials. If the pure thickness of a material is used for the weight given, it can be expected to demonstrate the qualities mentioned and to withstand the normal stresses of daily and sporting activities. Individual permutations on these figures will depend on clinical and technical skills

Patient's weight (1 kg = 1000 g = 2.205 lb, 14 lb = 1 st = 6.35 kg)	Category 1 Rigid material	Category 2 Semi-flexible material	Category 3 Accommodative material
	Rohadur	Subortholen Polypropylene Aquaplast Acrylonitrile butadine styrene	Ethylene vinyl acetate (measured in density of foam)
Less than 25 kg	2 mm	2 mm of Aquaplast for max. flexibility	220 kg/m³ Lower densities of polyethylene foam can be used if greater softness is required
More than 25 kg but Less than 45 kg	3 mm	3 mm	240 kg/m³
More than 45 kg but Less than 75 kg	4 mm	4 mm	260 kg/m³
More than 75 kg	5 mm	5 mm	300–360 kg/m³

From this chart it may be established that a person of 25 kg or less who is given an orthosis made of a 2 mm material from Catetory 2 will experience semi-flexible control. However, if the 'weight to thickness ratio' is now invoked and the same person is given an orthosis made from the same category of materials but of a 4 mm thickness, more rigid control of the foot will be achieved. This theory will also work in reverse, and with all the materials available, to develop numerous permutations.

The uses of these permutations are exciting. They allow the clinician wide scope in choosing the most suitable material for a patient's needs. The choice is critical to the results achieved. The following tables may facilitate the decision: Tables 2.2, 2.3, 2.4 and 2.5.

Table 2.2   Weight of patient—less than 25 kg

	Amount of joint control required		
	High	Medium	Low
S Rigid 2 mm H or E Semi-flex 4 mm (check L room in shoe and type L of activity)		Semi-flex 2 mm	Accommodative orthosis or Aquaplast
P Rear- O foot	360 EVA or acrylic	360 EVA	230 EVA
S T Fore- foot	260 EVA	220 EVA	220 EVA

Table 2.3   Weight of patient—less than 45 kg

	Amount of joint control required		
	High	Medium	Low
S Rigid 3 mm H or E Semi-flex 5 mm (check L room in shoe and type L of activity)		Semi-flex 3 mm or Rigid 2 mm	Semi-flex 2 mm or Accommodative orthosis
P Rear- O foot	360 EVA	360 Eva	260 EVA
S T Fore- foot	260 EVA	240 EVA	220 EVA

Table 2.4   Weight of patient—less than 75 kg

	Amount of joint control required		
	High	Medium	Low
S Rigid 4 mm H E L L		Semi-flex 4 mm or Rigid 3 mm	Semi-flex 3 mm or Accommodative orthosis
P Rear- O foot	Acrylic or 360 Eva with rigid insert	360 EVA	300 EVA
S T Fore- foot	360 EVA	260–300 EVA	260 EVA

Table 2.5 Weight of patient—more than 75 kg

	High	Amount of joint control required Medium	Low
S Rigid 5 mm **H** **E** **L** **L**		Semi-flex 5 mm or Rigid 3–4 mm	Semi-flex 3–4 mm or Accommodative orthosis
P Rear- Acrylic **O** foot **S**		Acrylic	360 EVA
T Fore- Acrylic foot		360 EVA	300 EVA

> Being in possession of the *exact* weight of the patient will enable 'fine tuning' of the weight/material ratio, for the best clinical results.

By following the 'weight to thickness' principle, it is possible to establish the qualities that the material chosen will exhibit under the stress of body weight during gait. It is now necessary to be able to relate these qualities to the use to which the material is to be put. Bear these thoughts in mind:

1. As already mentioned, the greater the rigidity of the material used, the greater is the control that will be achieved.

   However

2. a. If no range of motion (ROM) is evident in the joints of the lower limb associated with gait, then no control can be achieved. The material options here are limited to 'accommodative', in as much as they accommodate the deformity.
   b. If some range of motion exists, but is limited, the options vary:
      (i) If the joints of the foot are pain-free and/or it is desirable to increase the range of motion, then semi-flexible materials could be chosen.
      (ii) But if movement in the joints of the foot elicits pain, then control of available movement is desirable using more rigid shell materials accompanied by relatively soft post materials (with rigid inserts) to improve shock absorption at heel strike, together with cushioning covers to give comfort on full foot loading. This alternative is sometimes necessary, particularly in patients suffering from rheumatoid arthritis. In this condition where, so often, movement within the joints of the foot is very painful, the clinician is further hampered by a disease process which is constantly changing the shape of the foot. Skilful adaptation of the basic principles mentioned so far becomes necessary. The im-

pregnation and blending of controlling materials into accommodative materials will allow changes in shape to occur without reducing the functional properties of the device. Some time will be devoted to these adaptations later on.

c. In the child, control is required with sufficient flexibility to allow torsional adaptations. In treatments that are necessary to encourage the foot to develop more normally, semi-flexible materials are chosen.

d. In the athelete, it is important to know what sport is played and the grade. The types of sport vary as much as the materials used to control the foot during them. As a general rule, a person running large distances regularly requires the control of firmer materials. The jumper, on the other hand, who will pronate heavily into the device on take-off, requires more flexible materials.

The important factors that govern the choice of material may be summed up as *weight, activity*, the *aim of treatment* and the *range of motion* in the joints associated with gait.

As has been seen briefly, the decision regarding the choice of material for any given range of motion is made by evaluating the need for and

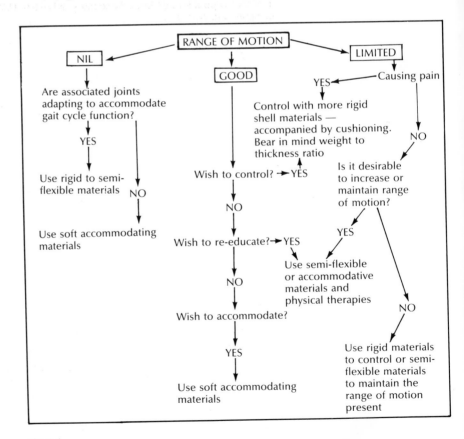

Fig. 2.1

possibility of gaining control,enlargement, or accommodation of the existing movement, or re-educating it. It is a clinical decision and is summed up in Figure 2.1.

SUMMARY

Four important areas of the decision process regarding material choice have been discussed. The rationale will now be developing to a stage where it is possible to relate:

1. The weight of the patient
2. The activity of the patient
3. The range of motion in the joints associated with gait
4. The use the finished orthosis is to be put to

} To the material of choice

NOTES

1. Wilh. Jul. Teufel, 7 Stuttgart 1, Postfach 1357, W. Germany.
2. Simona GMBH, Postfach 133, 6570 Kirn/Nahe.
3. WFR Corporation, 68 Birch St, Ramsey, NJ 07446, USA.
4. Smith and Nephew.

3

Negative cast creation and assessment

Once a decision has been made to go ahead with orthotic therapy, it becomes necessary to obtain a model of the foot to work on. This is usually done using plaster of Paris bandage.

PLASTER OF PARIS BANDAGE

Plaster of Paris bandage is a white cotton, open-weave bandage which has been impregnated with plaster of Paris. There are a number of these bandages on the market. Regardless of which brand name is chosen, however, it is important that the one selected is of low plaster loss (LPL). This means that an inert resin has been added to the bandage to help 'bind' the plaster of Paris powder to it, thus preventing the loss of the powder when it is immersed in water. The plaster of Paris bandage should also be rapid-setting, i.e. setting in 2–3 minutes.

The required length is cut from a roll of bandage. (It is important that it is not torn from the roll, as this results in a significant amount of the plaster of Paris powder being lost from the bandage.) Opposite ends of the length are held in either hand and the bandage is immersed in water. It will be noticed that many bubbles rise to the surface of the water at this stage. The bandage should be held under the water until the bubbling has ceased. The hands are then lifted from the water, the left hand first, in order to extend the plaster vertically over the container. The left hand is then lowered into the right hand, causing the bandage to concertina. This, together with a final squeezing of the bandage, removes the excess water, making the casting process significantly less messy. The bandage is then restored to its original length and held vertically. The right hand is released and brought up to meet the left, at which time the bandage is positioned between the thumb and index finger of the right hand. The thumb and finger are then slid down the bandage thus 'creaming' the plaster of Paris powder into the weave. This creates a smooth, superior finish to the inside surface of the resulting cast.

THE CAST

Three steps are necessary to produce a suitable cast on which to manufacture an orthosis:

1. Taking a 'negative' cast of the foot
2. Production of a 'positive' cast of the foot from the 'negative' cast
3. 'Modification' of the positive cast to allow for the weight-bearing tissue adaptations or positional changes desired.

THE NEGATIVE CAST

A 'negative' cast of a foot is a hollow mould taken by placing wet plaster of Paris bandage over the surface of the skin of the foot. Once hardened, this moulding is removed from the foot and results in the contours of the foot being reproduced. The cast used for the manufacture of a functional foot orthosis is known as a 'slipper cast'. It encompasses only the plantar surface and the medial and lateral sides of the foot to the height of the inferior surface of both malleoli. It is taken with the sub-talar joint in its neutral position and the mid-tarsal joint pronated and therefore fully 'locked' on the rear-foot.

TECHNIQUES USED TO OBTAIN A 'NEGATIVE' SLIPPER CAST OF THE FOOT WITH THE SUB-TALAR JOINT IN ITS NEUTRAL POSITION

THE ADULT

Materials necessary (per cast)

Approximately half a roll of plaster of Paris bandage (100 mm wide). (This depends on the size of the foot)
Two gauze swabs
Paper to cover the floor.

Tools/equipment

Rubber bowl
Scissors
Water-soluble 'fine' felt-tip pen.

Technique

1. The patient is lying prone throughout the casting procedure. A check is made to see if the heel bisection line marked on the posterior aspect of the calcaneus is clear. This line should be in a water-soluble felt pen as it will be vital for it to be transferred to the negative cast.

2. Position the posterior aspect of the calcaneus in the frontal plane. If necessary, this position can be achieved by raising the hip of the opposite leg. (This has the effect of internally rotating the limb being cast.) A folded towel is suitable for this purpose.

3. Cut out six strips of plaster of Paris bandage (100 × 400 mm) and arrange in two sets of three.

4. Place the two sets of strips on the foot while dry, so that they reach from the head of the first metatarsal to the head of the fifth metatarsal, one set by going around the posterior aspect of the heel and the other around the apices of the toes. They should overlap by 2 cm on both sides (Fig. 3.1).
   Cut off any excess.

5. Each set of three strips of plaster of Paris bandage is now treated as a single bandage. The first set is immersed in water, removed and the excess water squeezed out and the bandage creamed by the method described earlier.

6. Place the bandage on the foot from the head of the first metatarsal around the heel to the head of the fifth metatarsal (Fig. 3.2).

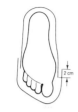

Fig. 3.1

Fig. 3.2

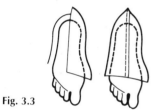

Fig. 3.3

7. Fold over one side just over the centre of the foot — then the other side, and close the seam (Fig. 3.3).

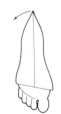

Fig. 3.4

8. The resulting tab at the top should be pushed away from the plantar surface of the foot on to the back of the heel (Fig. 3.4).

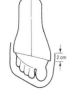

Fig. 3.5

9. Take the second set of plaster strips, immerse, squeeze and cream as before and place around the distal end of the toes, extending it around either side of the foot to overlap on either side with the plaster already applied. The overlap should be at least 2 cm (Fig. 3.5).

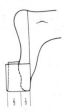

Fig. 3.6

10. Check that one-third only extends onto the dorsum of the foot and that two-thirds extends onto the plantar surface (Fig. 3.6).

Fig. 3.7

11. Fold one side over and then the other. Take the resulting tab and mould this into the webbing space beneath the toes (Fig. 3.7).
12. Now smooth the plaster well into the bandage, using the palm of the hand.
    Note: The time taken to reach this stage should not be more than 1.5 minutes, or the plaster will be setting before the sub-talar joint is positioned correctly.)

Fig. 3.8

13. Take a gauze square, fold it in half and place over the fourth and fifth metatarsal heads. This is an essential precaution to prevent the subsequent pressure from the thumb which 'locks' the mid-tarsal joint from disfiguring the cast (Fig. 3.8).
14. It is now necessary to position the foot so that the sub-talar joint is in its neutral position, i.e. if working on a right foot, feel for the head of the talus with your left hand, using your thumb on the medial side and your index finger on the lateral side.
    Press up on the fourth and fifth metatarsal heads with the thumb of the right hand until resistance is felt in the ankle. This will lock the mid-tarsal joint in its fully pronated position.
    (Reverse the hand position when working on the left foot.)
15. This position must be maintained while the plaster is setting. It is imperative that the patient is relaxed and the foot under the control of the operator. Any muscular contraction at this stage is certain to distort the cast, e.g. the contraction of tibialis anterior will result in an inverted cast.
16. Once the plaster has set, the cast is ready for removal. Gently ease the skin from the top edge of the cast.
17. The cast is now grasped at the top of the medial and lateral sides of the heel with one hand and across the metatarsal head area with the other. The posterior end of the cast is then pulled gently away from the heel, after which it is pushed downwards to free it from the foot (Fig. 3.9).
18. The cast must now be assessed for accuracy, to confirm that it concurs with the biomechanical examination results relating to the foot.

Fig. 3.9

THE CHILD (up to approximately 6 years of age)

The casting of a child's foot is inherently more difficult than the casting of an adult's. The reasons are obvious to anyone used to treating children. Apprehension and a short attention span on the part of the child, together with an eagerness to see what is going on, may lead to inaccuracies occurring in the casting technique described for the adult.

Furthermore, the child's foot is a floppy, mouldable structure, seldom restricted by the fixed deformities that must be compensated for in the adult. With children it is possible to correct the weight-bearing position of the foot while casting, to allow or assist its normal ontogenetic development.

Therefore, not only does the approach to casting need to be more subtle, but allowances must be made for the specific developmental requirements of skeletally immature infants.

Overall, a calm manner must be assumed, as well as a willingness to give the time necessary to make the child feel at home in a strange environment.

With calm efficiency and a modified casting technique, excellent results are sustainable.

Method

The child's foot is more profitably cast in a semi-weight-bearing position.

This method has a number of advantages. Firstly, it enables the correction of the weight-bearing position of the foot while casting.

Secondly, with the foot in contact with the ground, the child has a good view of what is happening and is therefore less prone to causing cast distortion due to fidgeting. Thirdly, the ground acts as a stabiliser for the foot and as a 'third' hand for you while casting.

Materials necessary (per cast)

Approximately one-third of a roll of plaster of Paris bandage (60 mm wide)
A 12 mm sheet of latex foam (150 × 100 mm) (A folded towel is a suitable substitute)
A plastic bag
Paper to cover floor.

Tools/equipment

Rubber bowl
Scissors
Water-soluble 'fine' felt-tip pen.

Technique

1. Be certain that a clear bisection line is present on the posterior aspect of the heel. This should be in a water-soluble 'fine' felt-tip pen.
2. Seat the child in a suitable chair that allows the foot to make light ground contact, with the leg at an approximate right angle to the

floor. The position of the foot at this stage is unimportant.

3. A piece of 12 mm latex foam should now be inserted in a plastic bag and placed under the foot. This will prevent the plantar contours of the foot from becoming destroyed in casting.

4. At this stage it is prudent to familiarise the child with the procedure to be performed. It also allows you time to visualise clearly the optimum functioning position of the foot. The criterion for this casting method is one of biomechanical normalcy. The easiest way to establish this in the infant is to observe the position of the talonavicular articulation and the position the navicular assumes within this. The foot and lower leg may need to be rotated transversely to achieve the correct position. The rotation is not important; what is, is the position of the navicular and the talus. There should be no anterolateral bulge of the head of the talus or antero-medial bulge of the navicular on the dorsal surface of the foot. Having positioned the foot to achieve the desired relationships, the leg is held (if working on the left foot) with the left hand, and the right hand is used to depress the fore-foot to make firm ground contact.

5. Having confidently achieved the desired position, the strips of plaster of Paris are cut to size, following the same criteria as for the adult.

6. The child's foot can now either be placed on a portable footrest or over your knee. The plaster strips are immersed in water and applied to the foot in a similar manner to the adult's.

7. The plaster is smoothed well and the foot is then returned to the position explained in Step 4. This position must be maintained until the plaster is set. The cast is then removed from the foot.

8. The cast must now be assessed for accuracy.

Note

An orthosis made from this biomechanically 'normal' cast only requires posting stabilisation at the rear-foot in order to prevent abnormal movement at the sub-talar joint. However, the anterior border of the shell must be shaped in the same way as is required when treating a foot in which a rigid plantar-flexed first ray is present (p. 159), i.e. scooped out to accommodate the head of the first metatarsal.

This is important in the immature growing foot, so as to encourage normal plantar-flexion of the first ray by peroneus longus which, in the closed kinetic chain, along with the plantar fascia, supinates the fore-foot at heel lift, thus locking the mid-tarsal joint and converting the foot into a rigid propulsive lever.

ASSESSMENT OF THE NEGATIVE CAST

Having taken a negative cast it is important to assess its resemblance to the casted foot. It must be an accurate reproduction.

Method

1. Rear-foot bisection line

The calcaneal bisection line drawn on the skin overlying the posterior aspect of the heel must have been faithfully transferred to the negative cast. If it is faint, it can be reinforced using a fine, water-soluble, felt-tip pen. If it is not evident or is unclear on the negative cast, it is essential to renew the line on the calcaneus and recast. This line is vital as a means of correctly angulating the orthosis during manufacture.

2. Frontal plane relationship of the fore-foot to the rear-foot

To examine this, the rear-foot bisection line must first be transferred to the outside of the cast.

The easiest way to achieve this is by shining a strong light inside the cast. If this is done on a freshly hardened cast, the rear-foot bisection line will be clearly seen through the cast. A straight-edge can be lined up with the image of this line on the outside of the cast, and a fresh line transposed. However, if a strong light is unavailable or for some reason the line is not clearly visible using the technique mentioned, two dressmaker's pins can be used to achieve the desired result, i.e. the cast should be positioned so that the fore-foot is facing the operator who then has a clear view of the rear-foot bisection line on the inside of the cast. One pin is pushed through the superior end of the bisection line and one through the inferior end. The cast is turned around to reveal the protruding pins on the outside of the heel. A straight-edge is lined up against these pins and a line drawn to join the two points, thus transferring the bisection line to the outside of the cast (Fig. 3.10).

It is now possible to examine the frontal plane relationship of the fore-foot to the rear-foot.

To do this the tractograph must be set at 90 degrees. One arm of it is placed upon a flat examination table and the other against the posterior surface of the cast. The cast is tilted until the rear-foot bisection line corresponds to the 90 degree angle set on the tractograph. It

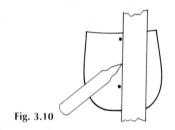

Fig. 3.10

RIGHT FOOT

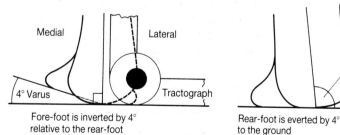

Medial　Lateral

4° Varus　Tractograph

Fore-foot is inverted by 4° relative to the rear-foot

4° eversion

Rear-foot is everted by 4° to the ground

Fig. 3.11

is possible at this stage to visualise if the fore-foot is angling in the way the clinical measurements suggest it should.

If the cast is released, allowing the fore-foot to drop to the table, the rear-foot bisection line should then correspond exactly to the number of degrees of fore-foot anomaly.

(Remember: the fore-foot angle is the number of degrees variance the fore-foot makes from a line perpendicular to the rear-foot bisection, i.e. 4 degrees of fore-foot inversion will result in 4 degrees of rear-foot eversion when the cast is standing at rest on the examination table (Fig. 3.11).)

3. Thumb print

The thumb print overlying the fourth and fifth metatarsal heads, created when pressure was applied to the foot to lock the mid-tarsal joint, should be examined:

    a. It should be shallow and uniform and accurately positioned

    b. It should not be surrounded by puckering of the soft tissues on its medial side. This may be an indication of an adductory force put upon the foot while casting, or an incorrect position of the thumb when casting (Fig. 3.12).

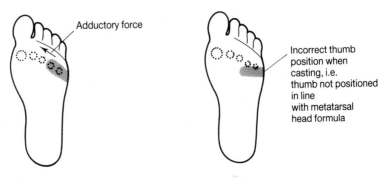

Fig. 3.12

4. Arches

The medial and lateral plantar aspects of the cast should be examined. If arches are present on the foot they should also be present on the cast. Furthermore, no creases should be evident along the extent of the medial arch, as these may be evidence of incorrect or insufficient loading of the mid-tarsal joint during casting.

5. Toes

The toes should not be dorsiflexed, plantar flexed, retracted or clawed on the cast unless they are so on the foot. Plaster of Paris bandage placed too tightly over the toes will cause this inaccuracy. It may also be caused by the patient being tense during casting and actively assisting the clinician at the time the mid-tarsal joint was loaded and the foot dorsiflexed.

6. Remember

A sign of any discrepancy relative to the casted foot should encourage the clinician to:

   a. Confirm the examination
   b. Recast the foot.

   Note: Patients who appear unable to relax during the casting procedure can be assisted by the administration of Entonox (nitrous oxide 50%, oxygen 50%).

4

Creation of a positive casted model of a foot

To manufacture a functional foot orthosis it is necessary to produce a strong 'positive' cast of the foot. This is done using fine plaster of Paris, which must be mixed very carefully if the strength requirement is to be achieved. A significant amount of pressure is necessary to mould a thermoplastic material over a cast. Nothing is more infuriating than for a positive cast to break under this pressure.

PLASTER OF PARIS

Plaster of Paris is a powder which is made from a crystallised mineral called gypsum. When this powder is added to water it will set in the exact shape of its container.

The chemical name of gypsum is calcium sulphate diyhdrate, which, when heated to 130° Celsius, loses its water of crystallisation and thus becomes calcium sulphate hemidydrate. This substance, ground into a fine powder, is known as plaster of Paris.

In use the powder is added to water, resulting in the reversal of the reaction and the reformation of the crystals of gypsum. It should be noted that this is a chemical reaction in which heat is generated and not simply a drying process. Therefore, if the powder to water ratio is incorrect, the gypsum will not be correctly reconstituted, resulting in a weak cast.

Points to note

1. Plaster of Paris must be stored in a dry place.
2. The handling of this material may cause an unpleasant drying of the skin. If this is experienced, rubber gloves should be worn.
3. Rubber bowls are required in which to mix plaster of Paris. Once any residue is dry, the bowl can simply be squeezed to crack the dry plaster away from the surface and aid in its removal.

4. Wet plaster of Paris spilt on clothing should be allowed to dry before cleaning is attempted. The dry plaster will simply crack and drop away from the garment.

METHOD OF MIXING

As mentioned, correct mixing of this material is vital if sufficient strength is to be achieved.

Powder to water ratio

It is difficult to be exact when quoting a ratio for the mixing of plaster of Paris because variations in the quality of the plaster can affect its mixing and setting properties. However, there is a method that seldom fails.

Method

Pour some cold water into a rubber mixing bowl. The amount of water needed can be accurately gauged by filling the negative cast with water and then pouring the contents into the rubber bowl. Having done this, gently pour the plaster of Paris powder onto the surface of the water until a conical mound appears above the water level and does not immediately sink in. (1 litre of water will absorb approximately 1.8 kg of good quality plaster of Paris powder.) The mixture is then stirred until it becomes thoroughly smooth and creamy. Care must be taken to ensure a total absence of lumps in the mixture.

The mixture begins to set just a few minutes after the water has been mixed with the plaster and is usually completely hard within half an hour. However, this setting time can depend on:

a. the quality of the plaster of Paris powder
b. the skill used in mixing—the more thorough the mixing the more quickly it will set
c. the temperature of the water—heat accelerates crystallisation
d. the rate of setting can also be accelerated by the addition of common salt. One teaspoonful to a foot cast is adequate to speed up the poorer quality plaster of Paris powder. However, fine quality dental powder sets quickly enough for most requirements. Having set, the plaster must be allowed to dry. The drying time may depend on the humidity of the surrounding air but can be reduced by the application of heat, together with adequate ventilation. Excessive heat must be avoided because a cast surface temperature of over 80° Celsius will reduce the final strength of the cast.

If the above principles of mixing plaster of Paris are followed, a cast of sufficient strength will be obtained.

OBTAINING THE POSITIVE CAST FROM A NEGATIVE CAST

Materials and equipment

Rubber bowl of sufficient size
Spatula
Sodium alginate cast-separating medium, or liquid detergent
Plaster of Paris powder
Water
Tractograph.

Method

1. The negative cast is checked for depth. If less than 6 cm is evident in all areas of the cast, some plaster of Paris bandage is made into strips and added to the superior margin on the negative cast. This is done to increase its depth and is allowed to set. The increased depth of the cast will help to prevent breakage when the thermoplastic is pressed.
2. Sodium alginate cast-separating medium, or liquid detergent (washing-up liquid) is poured into the negative cast and swilled around until it has totally covered all of the inside surface. The excess is poured from the cast, back into the container for further use and then the cast is allowed to stand upside down. This allows further drainage of the excess liquid and for the separating medium to dry without any 'pooling' that would otherwise occur in the plantar concavities of the cast.
3. Once the separating medium is dry, the heel bisection line on the inside of the cast is reinforced with felt-tip pen. Sufficient plaster of Paris is then mixed by the method already described.
4. A small amount of the liquid plaster of Paris is poured into the negative cast and swilled around the inside surface to produce a bubble-free lining to the cast. The remaining mixture is then poured into the negative cast. This must be done slowly, so as to prevent the formation of air bubbles.
5. The cast is then gently tapped with the fingers to remove any air bubbles.
6. The tractograph is set to the rear-foot angle that has previously been established, and the cast is positioned so that the rear-foot bisection line corresponds to this measurement. Ethylene vinyl acetate (EVA) off-cuts fashioned into wedges are suitable for propping up the cast. This process results in the upper surface of the positive cast being level once set, i.e. parallel to the weight-supporting surface when the rear-foot bisection line is angled at the rear-foot angle.
7. The cast is left undisturbed for at least half an hour to enable the plaster of Paris to set.
8. Once set, the plaster of Paris bandage is removed from the outside

of the positive cast. The rear-foot bisection line, if faint, is rein-forced.

9. The cast is now ready to be modified to allow for tissue adaptation on weight bearing.

5

The modification of a positive cast

This procedure involves a harmonious blend of technical skills together with a certain empathy for the foot and its comfort when wearing the orthosis. It requires as much artistic feeling as technique and takes thought and much practice to master.

Purpose of modification:

1. To remove the risk of blisters occurring in the medial arch by removing weight from this area.
2. To allow for tissue spread around the heel on weight bearing.
3. To enable the inevitable weight-bearing elongation of the cavus foot-type.
4. To allow the reduction of the lateral longitudinal arch enlarged by pronation. In feet where, on examination, an excessive supination is recognised at the mid-tarsal joint, often an excessive pronation at the sub-talar joint at mid-stance will result. In this compensated position an exaggerated lateral arch is recognised on weight bearing. If, with the patient standing, the sub-talar joint is returned to its neutral position, it will be noticed that the lateral arch disappears. Simply taking the cast in the 'neutral', non-weight-bearing position does not seem adequate compensatation for this variation in foot type. This must be accounted for in positive cast modification.

Materials and equipment

Tractograph or ruler with centimetre divisions
Pencil
Straight-edged spatula
Rubber bowl
Surform blade (convex shape)
Brightly coloured poster paint
Sanding gauze ('Sand-screen')—or wet and dry 180 grade sandpaper
Plaster of Paris powder.

Method

Filling the depression made by the thumb during casting

1. If the positive cast is dry, soak it well before attempting to add any additional plaster. As previously explained, plaster of Paris requires water to enable the regeneration of gypsum crystals. Therefore, if the positive cast is dry when additional plaster is added, it will absorb the water from the new plaster. This will result in a weak, poorly adhered modification which will shear from the cast under pressure.
2. Mix a small amount of plaster of Paris and allow it to set sufficiently to become the consistency of soft ice cream. Use this to fill the thumb print made while casting. Be careful to restore the normal convexity of this area of the plantar surface of the foot.
3. Allow this plaster to set and then use the Surform blade to smooth it to the shape required.

Marking out

The purpose of the next step is to mark lines on the cast that will indicate the borders of the shell of the orthosis.

4. *The anterior margin of the shell*

   This can be achieved in two ways:

   a. Place the positive cast upside down on the bench. Mark the plantar (sagittal) bisection of the first and fifth metatarsophalangeal joints in pencil. (It is sometimes easier to find these bisection points by first noting the transverse bisections of these joints on the medial and lateral sides of the foot. The marks are then transferred to the plantar surface, where the plantar (sagittal) bisection is made.) Mark these bisections with a cross. From the centre of the cross on the medial side a mark is made 1 cm proximally. On the lateral side, a mark is made 0.5 cm proximally. These two points are joined by a straight line which indicates the anterior border of the shell of the orthosis (Fig. 5.1).

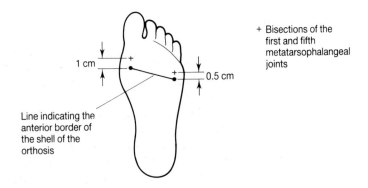

Fig. 5.1

b. The anterior border of the shell can also be achieved by another method should the bisection points of the metatarsophalangeal joints be hard to distinguish. Some powdered poster paint is rubbed over the bench top. The cast is positioned the right way up, with the plantar surface of the fore-foot sitting on the coloured surface of the bench. The cast is rubbed to and fro on this surface. When it is removed, a clear mark will have been made on the weight-bearing point of the medial plantar surface of the fore-foot. The central point of the mark is reinforced with a pencil dot. (Note: This is not a reliable way of indicating the lateral fore-foot weight-bearing point because the lateral arch is less pronounced and can cause smudging, resulting in an unclear impession.)

A mark is then made 1 cm proximal to this medial weight-bearing point. From this point, a line perpendicular to the long axis of the foot is drawn laterally across the cast. A point judged as the sagittal bisection of the fifth metatarsophalangeal joint is made on the lateral side of the plantar surface of the cast, 0.5 cm proximally from this line. This lateral point is then joined by a straight line to the mark made 1 cm proximal to the weight-bearing mark on the medial side of the foot (Fig. 5.2).

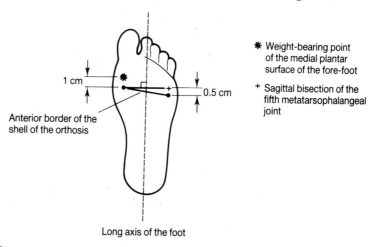

Fig. 5.2

The first and fifth metatarsophalangeal joint bisection marks, on the line denoting the anterior border of the shell of the orthosis, indicate the width of the orthosis at this point.

5. Heel cup

The heel cup must now be marked. The cast is placed the right way up on the edge of a bench top with the heel facing the operator. The medial and lateral posterior margins of the calcaneus are marked. The heel bisection line is positioned at the rear-foot angle decided by the clinical examination, and the cast is held in this position. A line parallel to the bench top is drawn on the posterior

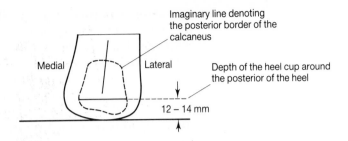

Fig. 5.3

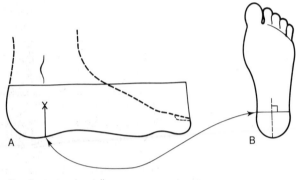

X = Sustentaculum tali

Fig. 5.4

aspect of the heel at a position 12–14 mm above the surface of the bench. (The choice of height will depend on the size of the convex curve of the soft tissues of the heel; if it is significant, the greater measurement is used.) The line extends, at the chosen height, around the medial and lateral aspects of the heel (Fig. 5.3).

6. A point corresponding to the sustentaculum tali is then marked on the medial side of the heel, and a line is drawn straight down from this point to meet the plantar surface of the heel (Fig. 5.4 A). The cast is then turned upside down and the line is continued, perpendicular to the longitudinal bisection of the heel, across to the lateral side (Fig. 5.4 B). It is then extended around to the lateral border of the foot cast, at which time it will meet up with the heel cup line already drawn around the heel. This line indicates the extent of the heel cup.

7. A mark between 5 and 10 mm above the line that was drawn around the back of the heel is made on the medial side of the heel on the line denoting the position of the sustentaculum tali. This point is joined to the posterior medial margin on the calcaneus, thus raising the medial side of the heel cup (Fig. 5.5).

   The choice of height at this point corresponds to the relative height of the medial arch.

8. *Medial and lateral margins of the shell*

   The cast is turned upside down once more and a straight edge is used to join the distal edges of the heel cup to the medial and lateral margins of the anterior border of the shell of the orthosis (i.e.

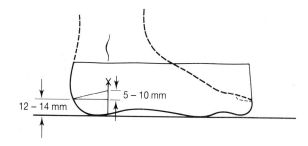

Fig. 5.5

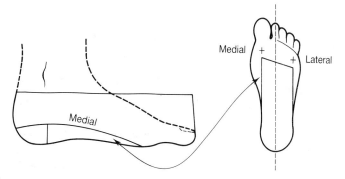

Fig. 5.6

the bisections of the first and fifth metatarsophalangeal joints). To do this, the straight edge will lean against the sides of the foot and cross at a slight angle to reach the points on the fore-foot (Fig. 5.6).

The lines indicating the borders of the shell of the orthosis are now complete. The next step is to add plaster to allow for tissue adaptations on weight-bearing.

PLASTER ADDITION

The practitioner with experience will move straight to this stage of cast modification, prior to 'marking out'. However, until a level of success and confidence has been achieved, it is wise to mark out prior to adding plaster, in order that the important 'landmarks' are clearly recognised.

The addition of plaster on certain areas of the cast enables the shell of the orthosis to be bent away from areas that serve no useful purpose in function and which often cause problems in use.

The areas where plaster is added are:

  a. the medial longitudinal arch
  b. the perimeter of the heel
  c. the lateral border of the foot.

Certain areas must *not* have plaster added to them:

(i) The plantar portion of a circular area of 2 cm in diameter, the centre of which is the junction of the superior medial margin of the heel cup and the line indicating the point of the sustentaculum tali. This area of the shell of the orthosis is relied upon to put significant pressure upon the foot, controlling excessive pronation at the sub-talar joint (Fig. 5.7).

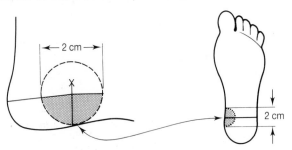

Fig. 5.7

(ii) On the medial side of the cast, 1–1.5 cm (depending on size of foot) proximal to the line made indicating the anterior border of the shell of the orthosis and lateral to the line indicating the medial side of the shell in this area (Fig. 5.8).

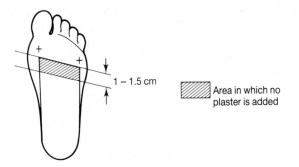

Fig. 5.8

(iii) On the lateral side of the cast, medially to the most plantar point on the convexity of this part of the sole of the foot (Fig. 5.9).

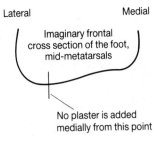

Fig. 5.9

SUMMARY OF AREAS TO AVOID IN PLASTER ADDITION

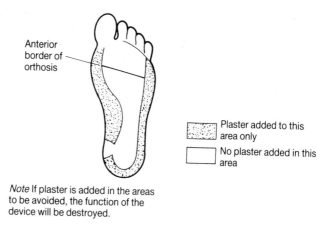

Anterior border of orthosis

Plaster added to this area only

No plaster added in this area

Note If plaster is added in the areas to be avoided, the function of the device will be destroyed.

Fig. 5.10

Method of plaster addition

1. The positive cast is immersed in water and left immersed during the next stage.
2. A small amount of plaster of Paris is mixed. However, before the powder is added to the water, the water is dyed by the addition of some poster paint. This allows clear visualisation of the additional plaster placed on the cast, reducing errors. The plaster is now allowed to set until it is the texture of soft ice-cream.
3. The cast is removed from the water and, if the operator is right-handed, it is held in the left hand with the heel facing the operator.
4. A spatula is dipped in plaster of Paris, which is then deposited on the lateral side of the cast as shown in Figure 5.11.

   The intention is to create a slightly flatter, wider shell of the orthosis. The process is continued until the lateral side and the perimeter of the heel have been added to. The shape that this process is intended to create is shown in Figure 5.12.

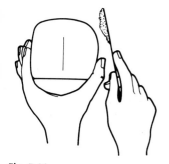

Fig. 5.11

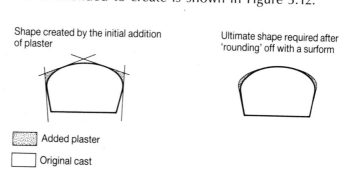

Shape created by the initial addition of plaster

Ultimate shape required after 'rounding' off with a surform

Added plaster

Original cast

Fig. 5.12

(Note how the convex shape is maintained but some allowance is made for the spreading of the soft tissues on weight bearing.)

Great care must be taken not to destroy the natural shape of the heel. This is responsible for 'cupping' the calcaneus and providing significant control during stance.

5. The medial longtudinal arch is now added to. A similar technique to that described in Step (4) is used. Figure 5.13 may be used as a reference to the area where plaster is added at this stage.

   Normally, not more than 1 cm in depth of plaster is added centrally on the most medial side of the cast. This becomes shallower and blends in as it travels laterally, proximally and distally (Fig. 5.14).

6. The shape intended for the medial arch (looking at an imaginary frontal cross-section) is shown in Figure 5.15.

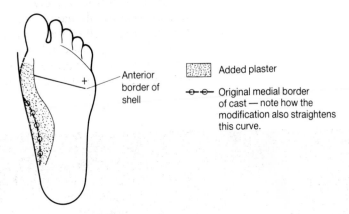

Anterior border of shell

⬚ Added plaster

–o–o– Original medial border of cast — note how the modification also straightens this curve.

Fig. 5.13

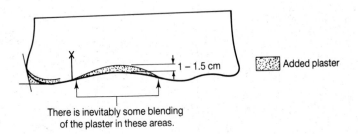

1 – 1.5 cm

⬚ Added plaster

There is inevitably some blending of the plaster in these areas.

Fig. 5.14

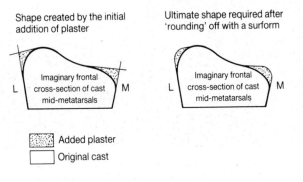

Shape created by the initial addition of plaster

Ultimate shape required after 'rounding' off with a surform

L   Imaginary frontal cross-section of cast mid-metatarsals   M

L   Imaginary frontal cross-section of cast mid-metatarsals   M

⬚ Added plaster

☐ Original cast

Fig. 5.15

7. Having added the plaster with a spatula, it is allowed to set before the ultimate shaping is attempted.

8. Once set, a convex Surform blade is used to grind the excess plaster away from the cast. Sandpaper is not used for the gross removal of plaster; it is inaccurate, producing an uneven surface.

9. Having obtained the exact shape required, Sand-Screen or sandpaper is used to create the final smoothness and to remove any mild serrations caused by the Surform blade.

10. Before it is possible to say that the cast is complete and ready for the next stage—manufacturing the orthosis—two things must be done:

    a. The top of the cast must be examined for total flatness both longitudinally and transversely. Any discrepancies must be removed to render it totally flat, otherwise it will break under pressure of forming the shell of the orthosis.

    This flatness is easily achieved by placing the cast upside down on a piece of wet Sand-Screen positioned on a flat surface. The cast is then rubbed to and fro until its top is totally flat.

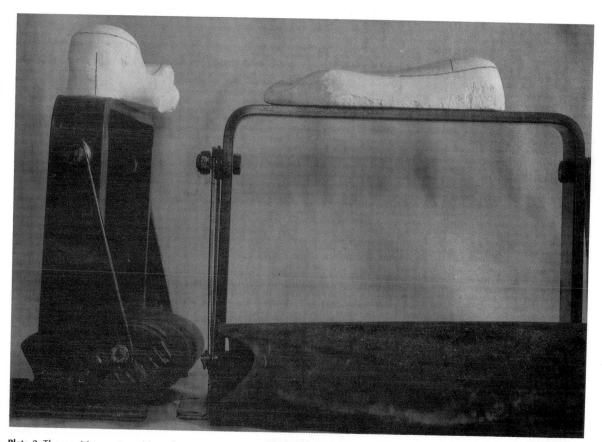

Plate 2 The positive cast positioned on a manual press. Note the totally flat surface of the cast resting on the platform of this press. This is essential if fracture of the cast during pressing is to be avoided. (© Enda McBride 1990)

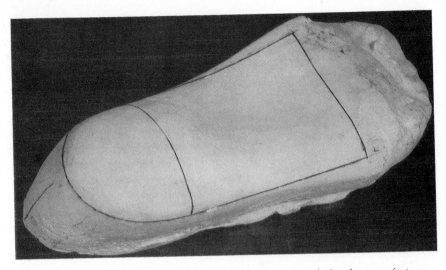

Plate 3 A positive cast correctly modified and marked out ready for the manufacture of an orthosis. (© Enda McBride 1990)

   b. If any of the lines drawn when marking out have become obscured when the plaster was added, they must be reinforced.
11. Once satisfied that the cast is totally suitable for the purpose, the next stage of orthosis manufacture may be attempted.

ADAPTING THE TECHNIQUE TO MEET SPECIFIC CASES

In this chapter I have attempted to explain a method of modifying a standard positive cast. However, in certain instances, there is a need to adapt the technique or to carry out some additional work before the cast is ready for the next stage of orthosis manufacture.
These instances are:

1. When the first ray is plantar-flexed
2. When prominences have been created by disfigurement, bursitis or nodules in the arthritic foot
3. When there are: the ulcerations that so often accompany peripheral vascular and arterial diseases; the wear and tear of physical ageing; and the neuropathies commonly seen in the feet of people suffering from diabetes, spina bifida, multiple sclerosis and leprosy
4. When there is navicular-cuneiform fault
5. When there are integral fore-foot extensions with EVA orthoses.

PLANTAR-FLEXED FIRST RAY

While this text does not attempt to teach the theories of biomechanics, I must stress the importance of the plantar-flexed first ray if the manufacture of orthoses is to be attempted. If this abnormal structural or functional position of the first ray is noticed on examination, a number of thoughts should spring to mind and be examined.

Firstly, the possibility of the fore-foot being in a valgus relationship relative to the rear-foot must be ruled out. It is, of course, possible that the fore-foot may assume this position and the first ray also be plantar-flexed. Whatever the case, the examination of the fore-foot must establish the exact neutral position of the first ray and, furthermore, its range of motion. If the first ray is plantar-flexed, then the knowledge of its range of motion from this neutral position is vital to the method of modifying the positive cast, let alone foot function.

The following situations commonly arise:

a. The first ray may be rigid and have no range of motion. The positive cast in this situation is modified as already explained in the text, and the first ray has no extra modification performed on it. The shell of the orthosis will later be modified slightly to accommodate this structural position and the fore-foot posted to prevent the functional adaptations.

b. The first ray may be mobile, but only with regard to dorsiflexion and this, to almost, but not quite the level of the other metatarsal heads. This situation is treated in a similar manner to (a).

c. The first ray is mobile and dorsiflexes to the level of the other metatarsal heads, but no further.

The cast of a foot with first ray motion such as this must, prior to the main marking out and modification being performed, have adjustments made to the plantar prominence caused by the first ray, i.e. when the negative cast of the foot is taken, the first ray will be captured in its neutral position which in this case is plantar-flexed. However, this is not the functional position. Therefore, the positive cast is ground down in the area of the first ray until the level of the ray and metatarsophalangeal joint are just slightly plantar-flexed, relative to the remainder of the metatarsophalangeal joints. It is important, from a logical point of view, to blend the reduction right down the first ray (metatarsal and cuneiform), and not simply remove plaster from the area around the first metatarsophalangeal joint (Fig. 5.16). Plaster must be removed the whole way down the first ray. Having made the adjustment to the cast to allow normal first ray function, it is then marked out and modified normally. In order to double check the functional position of the first ray, the relaxed calcaneal

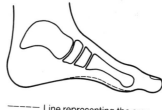

—————— Line representing the area
in which first ray is reduced

Fig. 5.16

stance measurement is taken to establish the effect the first ray is having on the foot at mid-stance.

d. The first ray is mobile and dorsiflexes past the level of the other metatarsal heads. If this motion is only marginally past the level of the other metatarsal heads, treat as in (c). However, if it dorsiflexes well past the other metatarsal heads, i.e. is hypermobile, the cast is ground down in the area of the first ray until all the metatarsal heads are in line and level, transversely. The cast is then marked out and modified normally.

Table 5.1 Summary of plantar-flexed first rays

Type	Rigid	Small ROM*	ROM to the level of the other four metatarsophalangeal joints	Hypermobile
Static level of first ray ------ Level to which first ray is reduced				
Modification instructions	No plaster removed	Treat as rigid, i.e. no plaster removed	Remove half of plantar-flexion from cast	Remove plaster to level of other metatarsal heads

*ROM = range of motion.   ⬏ = height to which the first metatarsal head dorsiflexes.

PROMINENCES AND ULCERATIONS

In the arthritic patient, prominences on the plantar surface of the foot, while palpable at rest, become more prominent and a source of much irritation on weight bearing. For these people and for those in which neuropathy has deadened the awareness of pain, such prominences not uncommonly ulcerate, jeopardising health and impeding mobility.

Areas on the foot that are affected by any of these conditions require enlargement on the positive cast, *prior* to the general cast modification and the pressing of the shell. This type of modification 'blows out' the shell in the area required and so totally relieves pressure and, it is hoped, discomfort. Because of what happens to the shell of the orthosis, I call this modification 'blowing out'. You will become familiar with this term as you proceed through the text.

In order that the position of the lesions and prominences may be enlarged accurately (this is so important), they must first be encircled on the foot prior to casting. A fine water-based felt-tip pen is useful for this. The areas must be reinforced on the negative cast after the cast separator had dried, prior to pouring the positive cast; this ensures accurate transfer. Once the positive cast has been produced, the areas of concern are enlarged by the addition of plaster of Paris. The enlargement must be done carefully and accurately; this will invariably amount to increasing the depth of the plaster by 4 mm.

The maximum depth is created at the centre of the lesion and is reduced by careful tapering, to reach the surface of the cast at a point approximately 2 mm wider than the actual border of the lesion drawn on the foot (Fig. 5.17).

Once these enlargements have been created, the cast is marked out and modified.

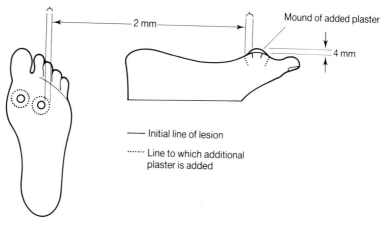

Fig. 5.17

Note

An orthosis or fore-foot extension pressed onto a cast modified in this way will reduce pressure in the areas that are 'blown out'. However, if it is also necessary to remove friction in the area of the metatarso-phalangeal joints, to eradicate damaging shear stress (as in the neuropathic foot), a rocker sole must be applied to the shoe. The ideal angle of toe-spring in this situation is 30 degrees.

NAVICULAR-CUNEIFORM FAULT

The long weak foot, in which this fault is recognised radiologically, requires supporting in the longitudinal arch, so as to prevent deterioration of the navicular and cuneiform and first metatarsal articulations.

It is important that a positive cast of this foot is not modified at all in the medial longitudinal arch, so that support is given to this area. In all other respects the modification is carried out as described.

INTEGRAL FORE-FOOT EXTENSIONS WITH EVA ORTHOSES

The method of cast adaptation needed in this instance is described in Technique II, in the chapter relating to the EVA orthosis.

Finally, do remember, when modifying the cast taken of the cavus foot, to note, prior to casting, the amount of elongation present in the foot on weight bearing. Additional plaster must be added to the medial and lateral plantar arches of the cast, when modifying, so as to prevent discomfort when the orthosis is being worn.

SUMMARY

Careful cast modification is fundamental to the comfort and therapeutic results of the orthosis. Owing to the individuality of every foot, it is impossible to cover here every eventuality that will arise. However, with clinical acumen, knowledge of the basic principles and the development of sound technical skills it will be possible to achieve good results in whatever situation presents itself.

> I often mention *thought* and make no apology for this, because it is always the vital ingredient to therapeutic success. For, if thought is given to each individual situation, bearing in mind the criteria mentioned and an empathy for comfort, a solution will be found; even if that solution does not reveal itself until the small hours of the night, when the tranquility of darkness sharpens true perspective. Study the foot, its structure and symptoms; study the cast, thinking all the time of the dynamics of movement, and think to yourself, 'If this were my foot, would what I am doing, be comfortable?' If the techniques are followed with this thought in mind, you will not go far wrong.

Possible alternative method using household filler

The cast modification explained in this chapter was performed using plaster of Paris. While this will be the most practical material for use in teaching schools, the individual practitioner may find a household filler, such as Polyfilla, more suitable. Although it is a little more expensive it does have certain advantages:

1. It can be mixed directly into a paste. This saves time that would otherwise be spent waiting for the plaster of Paris to set sufficiently.
2. It sets more slowly than plaster of Paris, giving a longer working time to perform the modification. The slower setting also means that more material can be mixed at any one time in preparation for the waiting casts. There is seldom wastage.
3. It smooths well once set, resulting in an excellent modification.

If a filler such as Polyfilla is used, some minor alterations to the technique described are required:

a. Because so little water is needed to render the material into a workable consistency, the colouring is best done by first dissolving the powdered poster paint in water. This solution can be stored in a bottle in quantity so that it is always ready for use. (Laundry 'blue' used as a colouring agent is a suitable substitute.)

b. The cast does not require soaking in water prior to modification, unless very dry.

c. The filler sets more slowly than plaster of Paris, which can cause delays. The setting time can be reduced by heating the modified cast in an oven or an old clothes-drying cabinet. Care should be taken not to raise the surface temperature of the cast above 80°Celsius, so as not to weaken it.

6

Materials used

THERMOPLASTICS

The enormous stress that a functional foot orthosis must endure has proved to be a stern test for many modern plastic materials. The requirements of high flexion and impact strength, together with the need for mouldability during manufacture, has limited the selection of materials available. Virtually all the materials used must be thermoplastic, i.e. become mouldable when heated. A number of the materials for functional foot orthoses are already in use for other orthopaedic purposes and meet the necessary specifications well. This chapter includes materials which at present are not commonly considered to be of medical significance. All the materials mentioned, if used according to the instructions and machined well, will produce an end-product that is comfortable and functionally enduring, as well as being pleasing to the eye.

ROHADUR

Rohadur is a strengthened acrylic which, although similar to Perspex in appearance, has, unlike Perspex, great impact and flexion strength. It has been used for orthopaedic purposes for some years and is ideally suited to the manufacture of foot orthoses when rigidity is required. Its general properties have already been described in the section dealing with the weight to thickness ratio.

Rohadur is orange in colour and sheet thicknesses of 2, 3, 4 and 5 mm are available.

It is softened by heating in an oven at 170° Celsius. The time the material takes to soften at this temperature is proportional to its thickness. When ready for use it has a rubbery texture.

Thickness (mm)	Time (minutes) taken to become mouldable
2	10
3	15
4	20
5	25

The heating time and temperature are critical. If Rohadur is not properly worked, the strength of the end-product is seriously compromised. It should be heated in an oven which is pre-heated to the required temperature prior to inserting the material. It is important that the material is not placed in a cold oven which is then allowed to heat up. This, along with fast cooling of the material (i.e. under cold water) or attempting to mould the material before it is sufficiently soft, will create considerable internal stresses and possibly minute stress fractures within it, which may result in fracture during use. Furthermore, great care should be taken not to overheat the material nor to maintain the working temperature too long as this will also weaken it. Overheating is indicated by a colour change from orange to dark red.

It is prudent to discard the material if stressing or weakening is suspected.

SUBORTHOLEN

Subortholen is a pressed, non-extruded polyethylene. It does not shrink when heated and can therefore be cut accurately prior to heating. It is flesh-coloured when cold but on reaching its moulding temperature becomes translucent. This property is a useful indicator. It is heated at 160° Celsius, the time taken to reach mouldability depending on the thickness. The time to thickness heating ratio follows closely that of Rohadur.

It is important that this material is not moulded onto damp positive casts. If this occurs, the surface of the material becomes pitted and disfigured. If time necessitates the use of damp casts, then they should be covered with a layer of tubular gauze or nylon hose material, as this reduces the risk of damage. The properties of this material have been described in the section dealing with the weight to thickness ratio.

POLYPROPYLENE NSR (Non-stress relieved)

'Non-stress relieved' polypropylene material exhibits great flexibility and impact strength. The colour is normally pale pink or white depending on the manufacturer. The properties are virtually identical to that of Subortholen and the heating temperature and times can be followed closely. However, unlike the materials already mentioned, it can also be heated under a small electric grill which reduces the heating time to a matter of 2 or 3 minutes.

It can be used as a substitute for Subortholen.

Note

It is critical that the 'non-stress relieved' polypropylene is obtained for the manufacture of functional foot orthoses rather than the 'stress relieved' counterpart. To look at they are the same, but the 'stress relieved' polypropylene will fracture in use. The distinguishing test is simple. The edge of a sheet of the material is held firmly between the jaws of a pair of pliers and bent. The non-stress relieved material will turn white along the line of stress, i.e. the bend line; the stress relieved equivalent will, however, demonstrate no noticeable change in colour.

ACRYLONITRILE BUTADIENE STYRENE (ABS)

Acrylonitrile butadiene styrene is a terpolymer which satisfies the requirements for functional foot orthoses admirably. While it is used primarily for injection moulding applications in industry, it is also produced in sheets of 3 and 4 mm thicknesses for the building trade and used as a wall-lining material. This material is also sometimes used to manufacture body supports and seat inserts for wheelchairs.

It is heated in an oven at 170° Celsius for 20 minutes at which time it becomes rubber-like in texture. At this temperature it moulds well but must be allowed to cool unaided to prevent shrinkage. It is a substitute for Subortholen and its uses are governed by the weight to thickness ratios mentioned earlier.

AQUAPLAST AND SANSPLINT

Aquaplast and Sansplint are low temperature thermoplastic materials sold in sheets. The 4 mm thickness is the only one of podiatric use. Orthotists use these materials to great advantage in splinting hands, particularly in the arthritic patient, as the materials can be applied directly to the skin. However, their use for foot orthoses is limited to children owing to their great flexibility under body weight. Therefore they are only advocated as a stop-gap when more suitable materials are unavailable.

Both materials soften when immersed in water at a temperature of 69° Celsius. Greater heat will not damage the materials but simply speed up the softening process. Aquaplast at this temperature turns from its cream colour to become translucent at which time it is ready to mould. Sansplint, however, demonstrates no change from its white colour and must be tested to establish its readiness for moulding. In general terms both materials take only a matter of minutes to become ready for use. Having reached moulding temperature, Aquaplast, in particular, becomes tacky. Therefore care must be taken to protect the positive cast by using nylon hose material. If this is not done, great difficulty will be experienced in removing the Aquaplast without destroying the cast in the process.

Furthermore, because of the low softening temperature of these materials, they will also become soft when being machined due to the heat created by friction. This disadvantage can be overcome by grinding in short bursts so as to prevent the build-up of too much heat. If use of these materials is intended, it would be advisable to acquire the pamphlet on their use, supplied by the manufacturers free of charge.

ETHYLENE VINYL ACETATE (EVA)

Ethylene vinyl acetate, a polyolefin co-polymer, is commonly known as EVA. It is manufactured in foamed sheet form primarily for the footwear industry, as a lightweight, shock-absorbing, hard wearing mid- and out-sole material. In my opinion, no other rubber substitute has been developed during my working life which, for podiatric application, has the therapeutic potential of EVA.

As well as being light in weight and shock absorbing, EVA can, in its lower densities, also be cushioning. It is thermoplastic, sticks with conventional contact adhesives, and machines well. If the weight to thickness and density ratio is used skilfully, the material has a useful life of approximately one year. It is also remarkably cheap to produce, and so if commercial considerations do not intervene enables the needy, yet financially less able patient to obtain suitable treatment.

It is available in foam densities of between 30 and 360 kg per cubic metre and in sheet thicknesses of between 3 and 12 mm. The heating temperature is 160° celsius, but the time taken for the material to become soft depends on its thickness and density. This, however, is between 3 and 5 minutes. A small amount of shrinkage will occur on heating, which should be allowed for. The material is used in the high densities for the 'posting' of shells of orthoses. It can be used in its full range of densities for the manufacture of 'all in one' orthoses. A whole chapter is devoted to these orthoses later, because the methods of manufacture and machining techniques are quite different to those of the other orthoses. The chart below relates the density of foams to their most common commercial use. This will enable a visualisation of the density prior to purchase. The densities I find useful are given in the chapter relating to the manufacture of EVA orthoses, and in the charts relating to the weight to thickness ratio in Chapter 2.

Common uses for EVA

Density (kg/m^3)	*Uses*
30–35	Soft buoyancy for lifejackets
	Sport protectors
75–85	Sport shoe insoles, sport protectors
140–180	Beach sandals
	Running shoe midsoles
190–220	Running shoe midsoles, casual shoe midsoles, slipper soles

220–300	Shoe soles for canvas shoes, lightweight walking shoes, bowling shoes, cricket boots, moccasins and slippers
300–360	Hard-wearing soling sheet with comparable durability to rubber microcell soling sheets.

DENTAL ACRYLIC

Dental acrylic was first introduced as a denture base in the early 1930s. It is a thermoplastic material, being moulded by injection methods under heat and pressure.

The method I use utilises the cold cure acrylic resin in the form of a liquid monomer and a powder polymer. It has a number of purposes in podiatry but can be used to advantage as a material for posting or stabilising the heels of orthoses. Methyl methacrylate is a liquid and is known as the monomer. If the monomer molecules are activated by heat, light or chemical, they join together to form larger molecules. The formation of these larger molecules results in the methyl methacrylate changing from a liquid to a solid, which is a polymer known as polymethyl methacrylate.

When the monomer and polymer are mixed together, two things take place:

a. The polymer particles dissolve
b. The monomer on reaching the polymer starts to polymerise.

This produces a dough-like substance. The rate at which the dough consistency develops will vary according to the temperature and the ratio of the mix.

It should be noted that the monomer is extremely volatile and the bottle should be kept corked and away from naked flames. Normal storage should be in dark-coloured bottles and away from the light. Since even a small trace of polymer will be sufficient to commence polymerisation of the monomer, care must be taken during mixing to avoid contamination. The polymerisation of the monomer is accompanied by a volumetric shrinkage of 10% and a considerable heat of reaction. This creates certain internal strains in the material during cooling. The effect of these strains can weaken the orthosis and cause warping, if the heat of the chemical reaction taking place during the curing rises above the softening point of the orthotic shell. When the high temperature thermoplastics are used this is not relevant, but it can occur when using a low-temperature thermoplastic for the orthotic shell, i.e. Aquaplast/Sansplint. The impact strength of acrylic resin is 4.2186×10^4 kg/m^2, or 60 lb per square inch. This has proved satisfactory for posting orthoses where it is used to obtain firm rear-foot control. However, because of its inflexibility it is most suited to application on rigid shell materials, i.e. Rohadur and 4/5 mm Subortholen (when this thickness of Subortholen is used as a rigid material). If used on flexible shell materials that may flex on the acrylic, the two materials may break away from each other during use.

It should also be noted that acrylic resin absorbs water (0.4% in 24 hours), which causes a slight expansion of the material. Furthermore, these resins are soluble in alcohol and methyl methacrylate. They must therefore not be allowed to come into contact with these solvents as the result will be a crazing of the surface of the material. The method of using this material will be described in the section on posting.

COVERING MATERIALS

Most orthoses require a top cover, not only for aesthetic appeal but, at times, to incorporate a cushioning material. Practically, there are three types of materials to choose from: leather, polyvinyl chloride (PVC) and 3–5 mm closed-cell foam rubber.

LEATHER

Conventionally, leather has been the covering material of choice. It is pleasant to touch, is unlikely to induce perspiration and sticks well to most materials. However, it is becoming increasingly expensive and the quality differs with the type of hide and the area of the animal from which it was taken. 'Persian lamb' leather reigns supreme for its flexibility, but is hard to come by and therefore calf skin is an adequate substitute. The 'cut' of leather best suited to podiatric use is known as 'top-split-grain'. This consists of the outside of the hide, or the part that has the hair on, which is known as the grain side, to approximately one-third its thickness (Fig. 6.1).

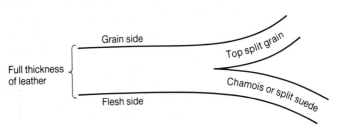

Fig. 6.1

The leather that remains from this splitting process is known as chamois, or split suede.

Generally, the leather most suited to our purpose, the most flexible, is found around the belly of the animal. This becomes progressively thicker as it proceeds to the back. Leather must be chosen carefully and is best selected by the potential user who has in mind the ultimate function required.

POLYVINYL CHLORIDE (PVC)

This material is commonly called vinyl and is manufactured in many forms. However, the forms with podiatric interest are those used for upholstery and flooring purposes.

The advantages of using vinyl covers for orthoses are many. It is consistent in its quality, is relatively cheap and can be washed to remove any soiling from everyday wear. However, it can increase perspiration of the foot and does not always stick as well as leather. This latter point is overcome by obtaining PVC with a cloth backing impregnated during manufacture. The backing provides a key for the glue.

The other PVC material of value is the 3 mm thick foam 'vinyl' floor covering. This material appears to contain a closed cell foam. It is actually manufactured in 'one run', the foaming process being curtailed as desired and sealed on both sides within a smoothed outer lining of PVC. Therefore the foam appears to be sandwiched between two layers of PVC. It is thin and durable and offers a practical solution to minor cushioning problems. As this material is unobtainable with a cloth backing, the side that is to be glued should be roughened well with sandpaper before being glued. If done thoroughly, good adhesion will be achieved. These materials are sold by the metre from rolls which are approximately 2 m wide.

CLOSED-CELL FOAM

Because of its structural make-up, closed cell foam compresses far less easily than open cell foam.

There are a number of closed cell foams available. Thickness of 3–5 mm are normally used and the one favoured because of its longevity, is 4 mm thick and is sold under the name of 'Spenco'. This has the added advantage of a nylon material already bonded to one of its surfaces, providing an aesthetic finish. Although this material is expensive in New Zealand, it is economical as it does not need to be replaced frequently. The use of these thicker foams is justified when added cushioning is required.

Open cell foam

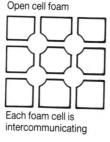

Each foam cell is
intercommunicating

Closed cell foam

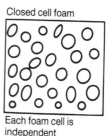

Each foam cell is
independent

Fig. 6.2 Cross-section of foam.

> *Note*
>
> Materials are constantly being updated and improved and so the preceding text is really a guide for the novice. Experience in the manufacture of orthoses, and sometimes the unavailability of the materials mentioned, will inevitably lead the practitioner to discover other materials which suit the purpose. This is to be encouraged, for it is the key to therapeutic advancement.

GENERAL PRINCIPLES OF WORKING WITH THERMOPLASTICS

SAFETY

Before starting work on plastic materials—*please*—for your own safety, consider these points.

High-speed electric grinding machines are potentially dangerous if sufficient care is not taken and respect given to them. A few small precautions will avoid the risk of injury:

- Long hair, if worn, should be tied back so that it is unable to fall forwards towards the grinding wheel during work.
- Neck ties should be removed, tucked into the shirt or fastened behind an overall.
- Loose-sleeved overalls should be avoided as the sleeve may contact the grinding wheel when the hands proceed forwards during grinding.
- Adjustments to the machine should *never* be made when it is running.

Remember

Plastics are noisy, dusty materials to machine. Goggles, ear protectors and face masks covering the mouth and nose *must* be worn. These are available from most hardware shops.

CUTTING AND PREPARING 'BLANKS'

A blank is a piece of plastic cut from the main sheet to the rough dimensions necessary to process it into the shell of an orthosis. If blanks are to be prepared in bulk, a measurement of 10 × 20 cm is an adequate size for the average adult foot (Fig. 6.3).

The bulk sheet must be marked out with a scribing tool. Pens should be avoided as they stain many plastics, thus compromising the final result.

The blanks should be cut from the bulk sheet using a fine-toothed (tooth pitch of 2–3 mm with only slight sets), fast running band-saw

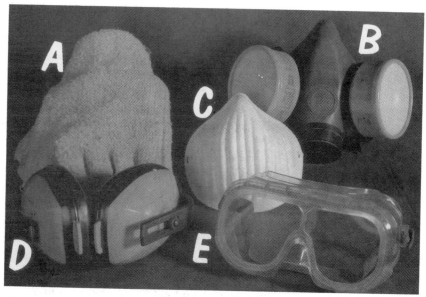

Plate 4 The essential personal safety equipment required when working with plastics. (A) Heat-resistant gloves for handling hot thermoplastic materials. (B) A face mask with replaceable filters for use when grinding and polishing thermoplastic materials. This type of mask is the most suitable. (C) A simple face mask to be worn if a mask similar to that shown in 'B' is unavailable. This mask should be close fitting and be changed regularly. It should be considered the *minimum* precaution that must be taken against the dangers of dust inhalation. (D) Hearing protectors. (E) Goggles. (© Enda McBride 1990)

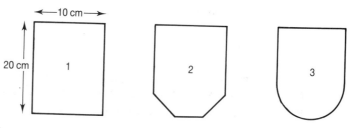

Fig. 6.3

(15–25 m/second). If this is not available, a hack-saw or jig-saw can be used. Failure to follow these cutting instructions when working with toughened acrylics will result in fine surface cracks occuring around the site of the saw cut. If these are not machined out fully, the strength of the material will be seriously reduced. When blanks have been cut to the size required it is wise to round off the corners of the end that will be ultimately pressed around the heel. This reduces the bulk and therefore the risk of buckling or puckering. As can be seen in Figure 6.3, this is done by cutting off the corners on the band-saw (2) and then smoothing the contour on the grinding, wheel (3).

HEATING

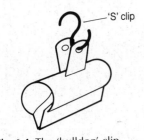

Fig. 6.4 The 'bulldog' clip.

Heat-resistant gloves must be worn when handling these plastics when hot. The heating of thermoplastics is ideally done in an oven which has a fan to circulate the air.

This type of oven is not essential but care must be taken to ensure even heating of the material. Small electric grills, except when mentioned, are unsatisfactory owing to uneven heat distribution. The most effective way of uniformly heating the material is to suspend it in the centre of the oven. A 'bulldog' clip is useful for this, if a piece of wire is bent in an 's' shape and hooked through one of the holes in the clip depresser. The other end of the 's' can be hooked over a bar of an oven shelf (Fig. 6.4).

The correct heating time must be strictly adhered to in order to prevent damaging the material and to ensure good moulding.

PRESSING/MOULDING

After heating a thermoplastic to the temperature required for moulding, it is formed to the shape required; this is called 'pressing'. It is not satisfactory to attempt to mould these plastics to shape by hand as great heat is involved, and quick even moulding is essential.

A press is required to mould thermoplastics. All presses consist of a flexible rubber sheet under which the positive cast is placed with the hot thermoplastic positioned for moulding.

The rubber sheet is then brought down on the plastic and stretched over it in order to mould it to the shape of the underlying cast. The two types of presses most commonly used are

—the vacuum press
—the manual press.

When using the vacuum press, the cast and plastic are positioned, the rubber sheet is brought down on it and secured with a clip. A vacuum pump is then turned on; as air is expelled, the ensuing vacuum pulls down the rubber and, in so doing, moulds the plastic to the cast.

With the manual press the rubber is forced down over the cast by hand. The end result is the same.

The press must be positioned immediately beside the heat source if possible. This facilitates quick transfer of the plastic to the press, which avoids the problem of cooling during transfer and thus a poor moulding.

When pressing plastics over a cast it is vital to ensure that the underside of the cast is *entirely* flat. If there is any unevenness either transversely or longitudinally, the significant force involved in pressing the plastic will break the plaster of Paris cast. The end result is also improved if the cast for pressing is covered with some discarded nylon hose material. This ensures a smooth shell after pressing and also prevents air pockets from forming between the cast and the thermoplastic during this process. Any air that would be potentially trapped is

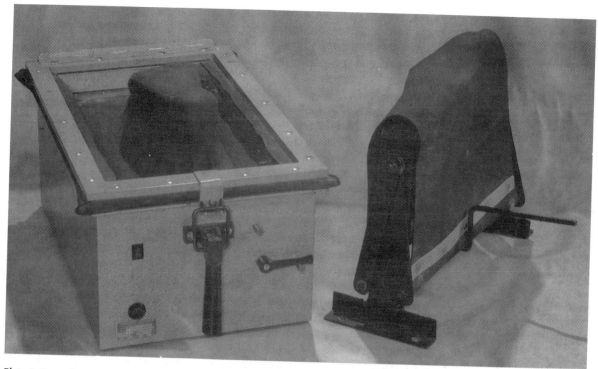

Plate 5 Examples of presses for moulding thermoplastic materials. An electric vacuum press (left), and a manual press (right). (© Enda McBride 1990)

able to escape through the meshwork of the hose thus preventing distortion. It is prudent to assist the moulding of the plastic around the heel of the orthosis with the hands to ensure good contact in this difficult area. Remember to wear gloves.

Having moulded the plastic it should be left in position under the press for at least 5 minutes, to allow the temperature to drop. It is then removed from the press and the shell is firmly bandaged to the cast until it is totally cool. This may take 1–1.5 hours. This prevents distortion and assures the perfect retention of shape. Remember not to attempt to aid the cooling process by means of a wet cloth as this can set up internal stresses in the material which may weaken it.

BEVELLING/GRINDING

(*Note:* The abrasiveness of sandpaper is inversely proportional to its grit number.)

A positive approach should be adopted when grinding and polishing plastics because small 'dabs' and careless angulation of the material on the grinding wheel leave uneven edges which may ruin the orthosis. Grade 60–100 abrasive paper on a motor-driven sanding drum is suitable for primary grinding. Ideally, a second drum fitted with an abrasive paper of between 150–200 grade should be used for a secondary grind-

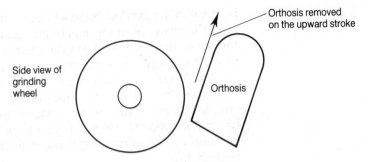

Side view of
grinding
wheel

Orthosis

Orthosis removed
on the upward stroke

Fig. 6.5

ing, as this removes any deep scratches and facilitates the polishing that will ultimately be required to achieve a suitable finish. Rohadur requires a final sanding, which can be done by hand under water using wet and dry sandpaper of 180 grade. The final sanding can also be achieved, with less effort, using pumice powder applied to a motor-driven cotton-mop polishing wheel which has first been dampened. The wheel must be frequently 'dressed' with the powder, which is itself best kept dampened and in paste form. (If a small dish is kept underneath the polishing wheel, then pumice, spinning off the wheel during use, is collected and can be recycled.)

The result required is one of perfect smoothness, as *any* scratch or

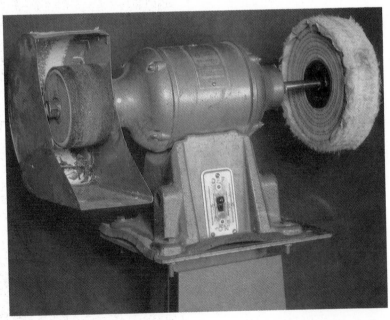

Plate 6 Grinding and polishing machines. Simple electric motors with the grinding and/or polishing wheels attached to the spindles are quite adequate and inexpensive. Dust extraction in this instance can be by way of a simple hood connected to a vacuum pump and waste bag. (A commercial vacuum cleaner is adequate.) The more sophisticated grinders are suited to a hospital, training centre or commercial situation—see Plate 7. (© Enda McBride 1990)

blemish in the sanded finish will become increasingly evident on polishing. The material being machined must not be held in one place for too long; the friction of grinding may cause sufficient heat to develop to melt the surface of the plastic being worked.

Furthermore, it is important that when grinding or polishing any plastic that the material is removed from the machine on the upward stroke (Fig. 6.5). This results in the waste material, created by the machining, being removed from the surface of the material as it is withdrawn. Do be careful if handling of the waste material is necessary; it will be extremely hot.

Specific details of the grinding techniques involved in the manufacture of semi-flexible, rigid and accommodative orthoses are given in the manufacturing instructions.

POLISHING

The finish on all materials is improved by polishing ground and sanded

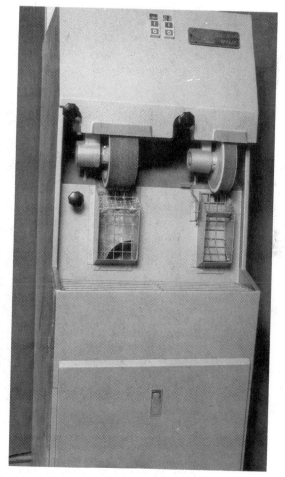

Plate 7 Heavy duty grinding machine. (© Enda McBride 1990)

edges on a motor-driven cotton-mop polishing wheel. On dense acrylics such as Rohadur, a superb glass-like finish can be obtained. It marks the culmination of your developing skills; for if technical perfection has been achieved in manufacture, great satisfaction will be derived developing the aesthetic finish.

For best results, two wheels are required. The first one should be 'dressed' with a suitable polishing compound.

The second wheel needs no 'dressing' and it is used to remove any traces of the polishing compound. This results in the production of a fine finish on the edges that have been worked.

The general principles of polishing follow closely those of grinding and more detailed information is given later.

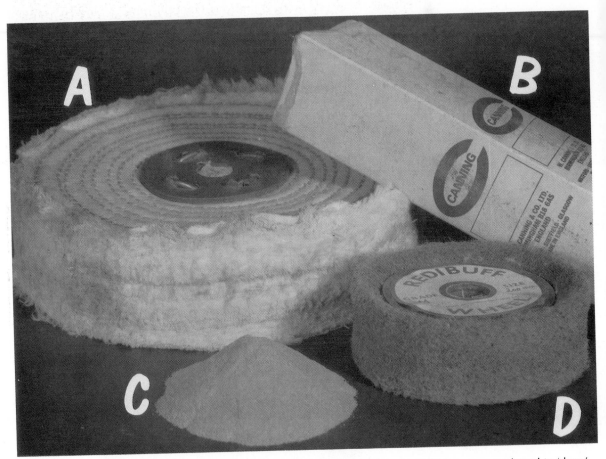

Plate 8 Polishing equipment and materials. (A) A cotton-mop polishing wheel. (B) Polishing compound used to 'dress' the cotton-mop wheel before polishing rigid and semi-flexible thermoplastics or acrylics. (C) Pumice powder. Used wet, this is ideal for smoothing acrylics after grinding. *Note*: A separate cotton-mop wheel must be retained for this purpose. (D) A Redibuff wheel, particularly useful for polishing polypropylene and the low temperature thermoplastics. Only light pressure is needed against this wheel. (© Enda McBride 1990)

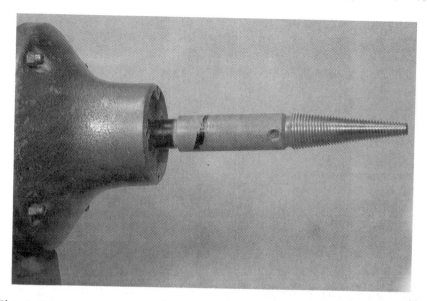

Plate 9 The tapered shaft. This attachment, when fitted to the spindle of an electric motor, facilitates the fitting and quick removal of cotton-mop polishing wheels. Be aware that a left-hand screw thread is required for the left-hand side of the motor spindle. (© Enda McBride 1990)

Note

Subortholen requires no polishing compound since the heat of polishing melts and smooths the surface. For all other plastics jeweller's rouge or borax paste is very satisfactory.

One general point

Cleanliness must become habit when making orthoses. It is disappointing to see a functionally sound device defaced by unnecessary glue marks. Therefore, masking tape should always be used to protect areas not being glued from the inevitable 'spread' that occurs. A little thought in this regard saves much time otherwise spent cleaning up and produces a more professional end product.

7

Manufacture of rigid and semi-flexible orthoses

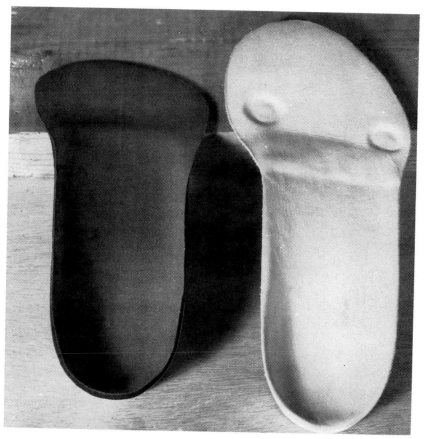

Plate 10 Two semi-flexible functional foot orthoses. The one on the left has a three-quarter length cover of Spenco rubber. The one one the right has an accommodative full-length fore-foot extension.

SHELL OF THE ORTHOSIS

The borders of the shell have been described under the section on marking out. It is the frame on to which will be attached the correcting posts, i.e. the intervening layer between the foot and the means of biomechanical correction. While playing a minor part in changing the angular relationships of the foot, the shell does, by means of its shape, enable the posts to work correctly. It is the part of the device that is in contact with the foot and therefore an indication to the patient of the measure of comfort and initial success of the therapy. Any biomechanical improvement will be worthless if, owing to poor workmanship, this intervening layer is itself uncomfortable. It must be machined carefully so as to remove any sharp, rough or thickened edges that may otherwise come into contact with and irritate the foot of the wearer, and it should therefore look and feel smooth to the hand of the machinist before being issued. Furthermore, the width dimensions mentioned earlier are critical, for if it is too wide it will be held by the shoe and compromise the desired foot function, while if it is too narrow it will be uncomfortable.

TECHNIQUE OF MANUFACTURE

The positive cast must be prepared as described, covered with nylon hose material, and placed upside down on the platform of the press with the heel facing the operator. A final check for any irregularities in the surface resting on the platform should be made and corrected if necessary. The thermoplastic blank is heated at the correct temperature for the required time and then removed from the oven and placed carefully on the plantar surface of the cast. It must be pressed over the cast *immediately*, as the working time is generally approximately 30 seconds.

Having lowered the press onto the bulk of the plastic, the heel area is given further assistance by cupping gloved hands around it. This ensures the accurate and complete moulding of this area. The plastic is then allowed to cool naturally and, if possible, while still positioned on the press. If this is not possible on account of the amount of work needing to be completed, the cast and shell can be removed and the shell bandaged to the cast using a crepe bandage. It is then allowed to cool while a further shell is pressed. Once cool, the shell is then ready to be cut to shape.

SHAPING THE SHELL

If the amount of material to be removed is excessive, the bulk can be reduced by using a band-saw. When using a band-saw to cut anything that is not entirely flat, thought must be given to the downward direction of travel of the saw blade (Fig. 7.1).

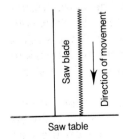

Saw blade

Direction of movement

Saw table

Fig. 7.1

With this direction of movement, these saws have the ability to pull the piece being worked towards them if it is not securely positioned on the saw table. When this happens, the operator's hands are at serious risk of being the first objects to come into contact with the blade (Fig. 7.2).

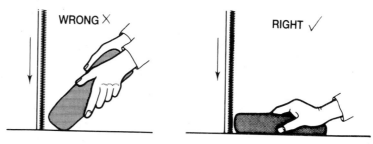

Fig. 7.2

Extreme caution must be exercised when using these tools. The work must be laid as flat as possible on the saw bench and held *firmly*. Care must also be taken to ensure that only one edge of the orthosis is being cut at any one time (Fig. 7.3).

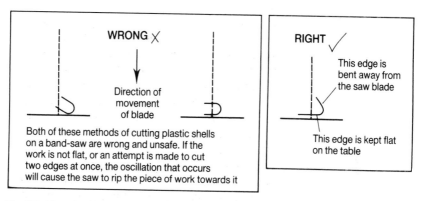

Fig. 7.3 View looking towards the cutting edge of the saw blade.

If at any time the work should show signs of being pulled towards the cutting edge of the saw *it should be released*. The work will invariably be destroyed by the saw but the hands will not be damaged.

When the bulk of the excess material has been removed, the shell is ready to be ground. During the grinding procedure care must be taken to make frequent checks to see that the lines drawn on the cast are being followed closely.

The first part to grind is the heel cup. To do this, the superior surface of the heel seat is presented to the grinder. It must be reduced until its superior margin corresponds exactly to the line on the cast (Fig. 7.4).

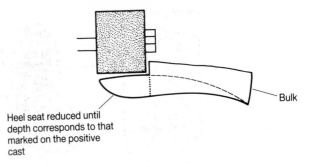

Heel seat reduced until
depth corresponds to that
marked on the positive
cast

Bulk

Fig. 7.4 View of the grinder from above.

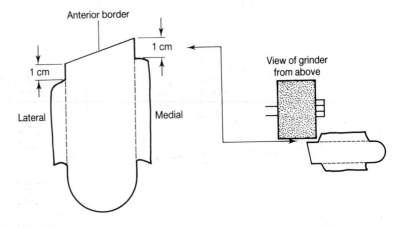

Anterior border

1 cm

1 cm

Lateral

Medial

View of grinder
from above

Fig. 7.5

The anterior border of the shell is then ground, followed by the medial and lateral anterior margins of the shell, which should be reduced to the necessary width 1 cm proximal to the anterior border (Fig. 7.5).

The bulk grinding is completed by connecting the medial and lateral anterior margins of the shell to the medial and lateral anterior margins of the heel cup. This is achieved by grinding each border independently, presenting its most superior aspect to the grinding wheel. Great care must be taken, particularly on the medial border, to maintain the straightness (longitudinally) of the border being ground, while also not destroying the sagittal convexity of the medial arch. This will be less likely to occur if the border being ground is uppermost on the grinding wheel. This allows a clear view of the surface being ground, enabling the convexity of the arch to be reproduced faithfully (Fig. 7.6).

Failure to have the surface being ground in the position mentioned, or grinding the medial and lateral sides of the shell with the heel of the orthosis uppermost, invariably results in the medial arch being 'ground out' owing to the inability to see the edge of the border being worked (Fig. 7.7). Grinding out the medial margin is the result of poor vision and excessive pressure.

With the exact shape now evident, the shell must be completed by taking away the edges that would otherwise cause discomfort. This is

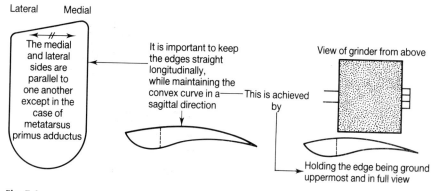

Lateral   Medial

The medial and lateral sides are parallel to one another except in the case of metatarsus primus adductus

It is important to keep the edges straight longitudinally, while maintaining the convex curve in a —— This is achieved sagittal direction by

View of grinder from above

Holding the edge being ground uppermost and in full view

Fig. 7.6

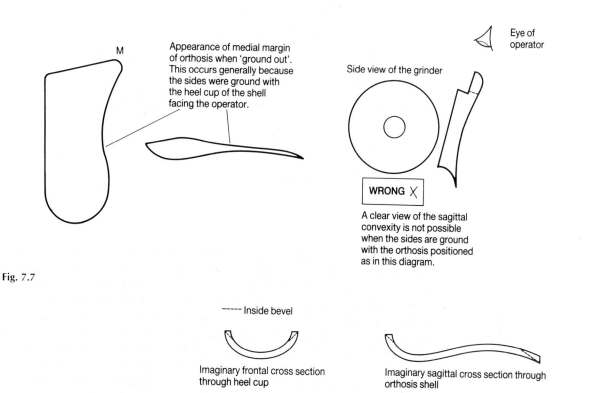

M

Appearance of medial margin of orthosis when 'ground out'. This occurs generally because the sides were ground with the heel cup of the shell facing the operator.

Eye of operator

Side view of the grinder

WRONG ✗

A clear view of the sagittal convexity is not possible when the sides are ground with the orthosis positioned as in this diagram.

Fig. 7.7

----- Inside bevel

Imaginary frontal cross section through heel cup

Imaginary sagittal cross section through orthosis shell

Fig. 7.8

done by producing a 'top bevel' or inside bevel on the inside of all the superior borders of the shell (Fig. 7.8) i.e. the heel cup, the medial and lateral borders and the anterior border.

This bevel must develop into a blending of the margins and it requires some 'feeling' for the foot of the wearer, as much as anything else. If an outside bevel is attempted, a sharp edge will be created at the superior border of the shell of the orthosis. This may cause discomfort if the soft tissues around the heel should bulge slightly over. Half of the thickness of the shell material ground on the inside and

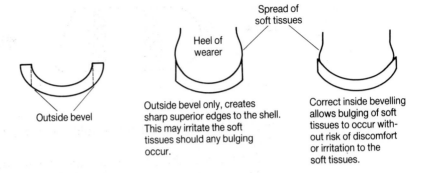

Spread of
soft tissues

Heel of
wearer

Outside bevel

Outside bevel only, creates
sharp superior edges to the shell.
This may irritate the soft
tissues should any bulging
occur.

Correct inside bevelling
allows bulging of soft
tissues to occur with-
out risk of discomfort
or irritation to the
soft tissues.

Fig. 7.9

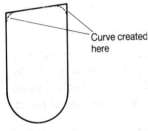

Curve created
here

Fig. 7.10

half on the outside is a worthwhile compromise if room in the shoe
around the heel cup is limited (Fig. 7.9).

Finally, a curve is created on the medial and lateral sides of the
anterior border of the shell, as shown in Figure 7.10. The shell may
now be polished.

POLISHING THE SHELL

The shell can now be polished using a cotton-mop polishing wheel
which has been 'dressed' with plastic polishing compound. However,
if polishing Rohadur, *all* the scratches produced while grinding must
be removed prior to polishing. This is achieved using 180 grit wet and
dry sandpaper and sanding under cold water, or by using pumice powder, as has already been described. Any mark that is left will be evident when polishing is attempted. All the other materials may be
polished immediately after machine-grinding. Polishing is best achieved
using short firm strokes on the wheel, as this prevents the polishing
wheel from producing excessive heat which could soften and distort
the plastic. Care should also be taken to remove the work on the upward stroke as this removes any debris, leaving the work clean. The
polishing of Rohadur is complete when a high shine has been achieved.
The polishing of Subortholen, Polyproylene NSR, ABS, Aquaplast and
Sansplint results in a smooth surface but only a dull shine.

PREPARATION FOR THE 'POSTING' OF THE SHELL

Cleanliness is of paramount importance when attempting this next step
in the manufacture of the orthosis. The posting material requires to be
attached to the surface of the shell using a 'contact' adhesive. It is prudent for the operator to use masking tape to protect the areas not re-
quiring glue from the cosmetic damage that will result from an
over-zelous use of the glue brush.

Masking tape is therefore applied to the shell at the distal margin of
the heel post (Fig. 7.13) and the proximal margin of the fore-foot post

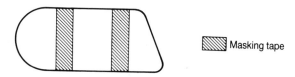

Fig. 7.11

(Fig. 7.30). It is placed perpendicular to the long axis of the heel (Fig. 7.11).

The areas of the shell which are to have the posting material stuck to them are roughened using 180 grit sandpaper.

CONTACT ADHESIVE

There are many brands of these adhesives available, all containing a rubber-based adhesive kept in a liquid state during storage by a volatile inflammable solvent. The solvent releases a toxic vapour which should not be inhaled. It should therefore be used in a well-ventilated room and kept away from naked flames.

To use this glue, a thin layer should be spread upon both the surfaces that are to be stuck to one another. A 25 mm paint-brush is ideal for this, which after use is placed in a tightly capped jar containing the correct solvent for the brand of adhesive being used. This prevents the glue from drying and ruining the brush. The adhesive spread onto the materials that are to be stuck together is allowed to become 'touch' dry. This takes approximately 10 to 15 minutes, after which the two surfaces are brought into contact with one another. Adhesion is immediate. This necessitates accurate placement, as it is not possible to 'slip' the surfaces upon one another. Heat and pressure will improve adhesion.

POSTING

The principle involved in posting is to prevent pathological compensation in a biomechanically abnormal and inefficient limb. Such a limb is subjected to undue stress owing to the greater degrees of motion required to function as a stable support and propellant during the gait cycle. By 'posting' the foot, the clinician endeavours to alter the position of the supporting surface on which the limb is functioning and by careful analysis bring it into contact with the foot at the correct moment during the gait cycle. In controlling the sub-talar and mid-tarsal joints by raising the ground to meet the plantar surface of the foot, unnecessary compensatory movement is prevented and symptoms associated with it relieved.

For example, a foot that is supinated at the fore-foot relative to the rear-foot will place demands upon the sub-talar joint which this joint

Representation of a foot with the sub-talar joint in neutral and the fore-foot relatively supinated

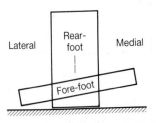

In order that the fore-foot can make ground-contact the calcaneus must evert excessively

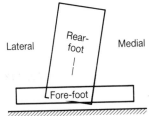

By controlling the calcaneus and fore-foot with 'posts' the compensatory eversion of the calcaneus is prevented

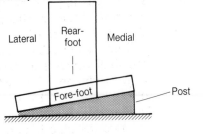

Fig. 7.12 Diagrammatic impression of rear-foot and fore-foot.

may be unable to accommodate. Any manner of positional and functional changes may occur in the affected limb to compensate for this anomaly. By controlling the movement in the sub-talar joint and raising the ground to meet the fore-foot, the need for compensation is removed and the limb is able to function normally (Fig. 7.12).

It is a simple concept yet one that demands skilled clinical interpretation to execute successfully.

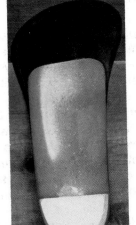

Plate 11 The underside of an orthosis, showing the rear-foot post.

REAR-FOOT POST

The rear-foot or heel post is applied to the shell of the orthosis in an effort to control the positional relationship of the articular facets of the sub-talar joint at mid-stance. It encompasses the heel cup of the shell with its anterior border lying 1 cm proximal to the transverse line drawn on the positive cast from the sustentaculum tali around to the lateral border (Fig. 7.13).

This post is always applied and machined first. The choice of material is a clinical decision, but the two practical choices at the time of writing are:

    a. Ethylene vinyl acetate with or without rigid inserts
    b. Dental acrylic.

Ethylene vinyl acetate

The material in the density of choice is cut to size using a sharp knife

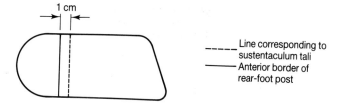

Fig. 7.13

or band saw. Fourteen millimetres is the average thickness required. When this material is heated there will be a small amount of linear shrinkage (approximately 4 mm) which should be allowed for. The anterior border of this post is machined totally straight. This must be done before adhesion, as any attempt to do so once the post is stuck will invariably cause damage to the shell of the orthosis. The area of the shell which is to have the posting material stuck to it is roughened with sandpaper. Contact adhesive is then applied to the correct area of the shell and to the EVA posting material and allowed to become touch dry.

Once the glue is dry, the EVA is placed, glue side uppermost, in an oven at the correct temperature for approximately 4 minutes. During this time the shell of the orthosis is placed upon the positive cast, which is positioned upside down on the pressing platform. The heated EVA is removed from the oven and immediately positioned on the shell, at which time it is pressed and allowed to cool under pressure.

It is then necessary to angle the heel post correctly to achieve the desired sub-talar joint function. This is achieved by careful grinding.

GRINDING THE REQUIRED ANGLE ONTO A REAR-FOOT POST

The shell is placed upon the positive cast and fixed securely by means of masking tape which encircles the shell and the cast. This prevents the occurrence of any movement which may lead to inaccuracies. With the shell and the cast securely fixed to one another, the tractograph is set at the frontal plane rear-foot angle required.

It is important at this stage to note the height of heel worn by the person for whom the orthosis is to be made. This is for a good reason as often the height of the heel worn by the two sexes differs. If no allowance is made for the differing heel heights, or any heel height at all, undue stress will be placed upon the shell of the orthosis and result in fracture. The reason becomes clear if the examples given below are examined (Fig. 7.14).

The average heel allowance that appears adequate is 4 mm for men and 6 mm for women; however, the heel height of individual patients should always be checked.

An off-cut of EVA makes a suitable platform to raise the heel while marking out prior to grinding.

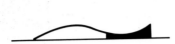

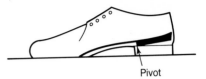

Pivot

1. Rear-foot post machined so that its full longitudinal surface is in ground contact when the supporting surface is flat.

2. The same orthosis put in a heeled shoe will pivot on the distal border of the post, compromising function and comfort and placing undue strain on the shell material.

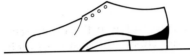

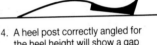

3. An allowance must be made on the distal border of the heel post to allow for the heel height.

4. A heel post correctly angled for the heel height will show a gap between its anterior edge and the supporting surface when this surface is flat.

Fig. 7.14

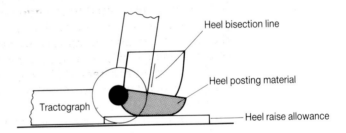

Heel bisection line

Heel posting material

Tractograph

Heel raise allowance

Fig. 7.15

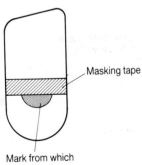

Masking tape

Mark from which grinding must begin

Fig. 7.16

Having set the tractograph to the required frontal plane measurement, the heel post of the orthosis is placed on the heel height of choice. The piece of material used to raise the heel must be covered on its superior surface by a light dusting of powdered poster paint or talcum powder.

The operator then stands behind the orthosis so that a clear view of the rear-foot bisection line is available. The heel is angled in the frontal plane so that this line corresponds to the edge of the tractograph, which has been correctly angled (Fig. 7.15).

The cast, shell and post are gently rubbed forwards and backwards on the material used to raise the heel, taking care not to alter the frontal plane angulation. This procedure results in a mark being made on the under surface of the heel post, indicating the point at which the machining of the post must begin (Fig. 7.16).

This mark will be noticed as being, on average, approximately 1–1.5 cm in diameter. An attempt should be made to present this marked area of the post to the grinding machine, so that the two outer edges

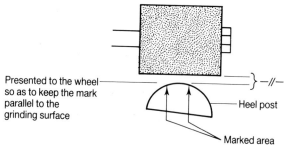

Presented to the wheel so as to keep the mark parallel to the grinding surface

Heel post

Marked area

Fig. 7.17 View of grinder from above.

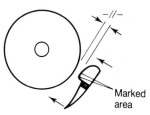

Marked area

Fig. 7.18 Side view of grinder.

of the mark are parallel in the transverse plane to the abrasive surface of the grinding wheel. This is necessary in order to develop the correct frontal plane angulation of the rear-foot post (Fig. 7.17).

Next, to achieve the correct longitudinal angulation of the orthosis, the centre of the marked area should be positioned so as to be the first part of the area to come into contact with the grinding wheel (Fig. 7.18).

To do this, the operator must be comfortable and in a position that allows a clear view of the work being machined. This is best achieved if the work is presented to the grinder with the longitudinal axis of the powdered paint mark parallel to an imaginary line running perpendicular to a line positioned approximately 10 degrees below the centre of the working surface of the grinding wheel (Fig. 7.19).

After this start has been achieved, even pressure both transversly and longitudinally is required to maintain accuracy. Unfortunately, it is not possible to hold the post in one place on the grinding wheel or a concave grind will be achieved (Fig. 7.20).

The work must be moved up and down the wheel in order to render flat the inferior surface of the post. The movement must be straight and along the imaginary line already mentioned, which is perpendicular to a line positioned approximately 10 degrees below the centre of the grinding wheel. This movement is consistently possible if the upper arms are held firmly locked against the chest and the wrists perfectly

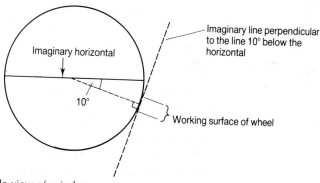

Imaginary horizontal

Imaginary line perpendicular to the line 10° below the horizontal

10°

Working surface of wheel

Fig. 7.19 Side view of grinder.

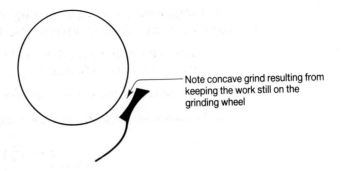

Note concave grind resulting from keeping the work still on the grinding wheel

Fig. 7.20

Imaginary guide lines which should always be kept in your mind

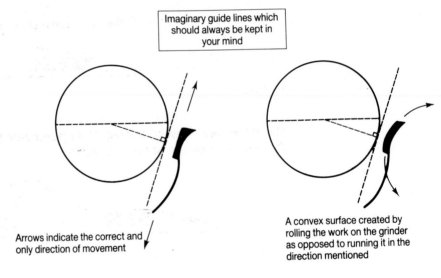

Arrows indicate the correct and only direction of movement

A convex surface created by rolling the work on the grinder as opposed to running it in the direction mentioned

Fig. 7.21

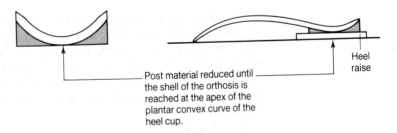

Post material reduced until the shell of the orthosis is reached at the apex of the plantar convex curve of the heel cup.

Heel raise

Fig. 7.22

still. The only movement that should occur is at the elbows and in a slight drop of the shoulders as the work proceeds downwards. Any rocking of the hands or arms will result in a convex inferior surface to the post which is totally useless (Fig. 7.21).

The grinding of the platform of this post is complete when the material has been reduced to the level of the shell material at its lowest point, i.e. the apex of the plantar curve of the heel cup (Fig. 7.22).

It is important to check constantly the progress of the grinding to assess accuracy. Once completed, the heel post should:

1. Have been ground until it has been reduced to the level of the shell material as indicated (Fig. 7.22).

And when raised to the correct heel height should be—

2. In total contact with the heel raise longitudinally (Fig. 7.23)

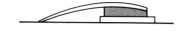

Fig. 7.23

3. In total contact with the heel raise transversely (Fig. 7.24)

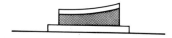

Fig. 7.24

The heel post is then tapered at its perimeter to allow a snug fit into the heel-seat of the shoe (Fig. 7.25).

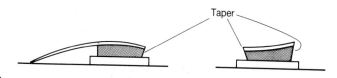

Fig. 7.25

REINFORCING THE MEDIAL SIDE OF THE HEEL POST

If it was thought therapeutically advantageous to use less dense EVA to post the heel of the orthosis, to allow some shock absorption at heel strike, or if the degree of correction is so large as to put a severe pronatory force on the post, thus risking premature medial distortion of the material, it is now necessary to insert a denser material on the medial side of the post to increase function. This can be done by the insertion of either:

Nylon screws
Epoxy resin
Dental acrylic
Wooden dowelling.

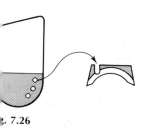

Technique

Having ground the heel post to the required angle and tapered the perimeter, three holes are drilled through the material to the depth of two-thirds of the shell (Fig. 7.26).

7.26

If nylon screws are used, they can now be screwed into these holes. If these are unavailable, wooden dowelling can be stuck into the holes, or epoxy resin or dental acrylic can be mixed up and poured into the holes and allowed to set. Any excess material protruding from the surface of the heel post should be ground away when set to render the surface flat. Once the operation is complete, a piece of 1 mm polypropylene or 1 mm fibre-board is stuck over the whole surface of the post. This avoids any risk of detachment of the reinforcing material during use.

THE FORE-FOOT POST

The decision to apply and the angle to which the fore-foot post is ground is a little more complex than that regarding the rear-foot post, which corresponds to the rear-foot angle. The decision in this instance depends on a number of things.

1. The age of the patient. The flexible deformities of the child will have been allowed for in the casting procedure, which created biomechanical normalcy thus negating the need for fore-foot posting. A rear-foot post in this instance is sufficient to control sub-talar joint motion. It is in the rigid deformities of the adult that the following considerations must be taken into account.
2. Is the fore-foot anomaly valgus or varus? In valgus anomalies of the fore-foot it is generally the unlocking of the mid-tarsal joint at mid-stance that this deformity allows, which creates problems associated with this foot type. The posting of the fore-foot in this situation is absolute. In varus deformities of the fore-foot the decision regarding the degree of posting is a little more complex and is governed by the range of motion at the sub-talar joint and the need for normal sub-talar joint motion.

The normal motion at the sub-talar joint requires it to pronate by approximately 4 degrees at mid-stance. Therefore if we examine this literally and if the range of motion is normal, 4 degrees must be deducted from the fore-foot angle to allow the orthosis to rock and allow this normal motion at mid-stance. It also then follows that if the fore-foot angle is 4 degrees or less, no fore-foot posting is added.

> i.e. Rear-foot angle = 4 degrees varus—post to 4 degrees varus
> Fore-foot angle = 7 degrees varus—post to 3 degrees varus
> *or* Rear-foot angle = 4 degrees varus—post to 4 degrees varus
> Fore-foot angle = 4 degrees varus—no post added.

However, if the range of motion at the sub-talar joint is limited or non-existent, the posting will increase nearer to the pure fore-foot angle, depending on the range of motion available.

It is inversely proportional. This reduction of the fore-foot angle, to produce the correct degree of fore-foot posting, is the *true* amount necessary to allow normal sub-talar joint function. However, technically,

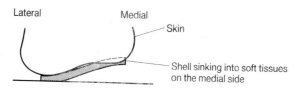

Fig. 7.27

one other factor comes into play. This is the thickness of the material used to make the shell of the orthosis. It is safe to say that if the material used is 4 mm thick or more, 2 degrees only are deducted from the fore-foot posting angle. This is confusing but is technically necessary owing to the lift this thickness of material gives to the lateral side of the fore-foot. If 4 degrees are deducted from the fore-foot post when using this thickness of material, the amount of pronatory tilt is too great and the symptoms the patient presents with are unlikely to resolve (Fig. 7.27).

The lift is due to the lesser amount of soft tissue present on the lateral side of the foot proximal to the metatarsal head as compared to the medial side. This causes the shell to be proud of the foot on the lateral side while sinking in slightly on the medial side. The overall result of this technical detail is to increase the height of the foot from the ground on the lateral side.

SUMMARY OF POSTING TECHNIQUE

- The rear-foot post is absolute, i.e. equal to the rear-foot angle except in the instance mentioned in Chapter 1.
- The fore-foot post, if using shell materials up to 3 mm in thickness and if the range of motion at the sub-talar joint is normal, corresponds to the fore-foot angle *minus* 4 degrees to allow normal motion at the sub-talar joint. If the shell material is of 4 mm or more in thickness, then only 2 degrees are deducted from the fore-foot angle.
- If the range of motion at the sub-talar joint is limited or non-existent, then the fore-foot post corresponds more closely to the pure fore-foot angle depending on the degrees of motion available.
- When normal motion is available at the sub-talar joint, then preventing pronation by absolute posting not only prevents normal foot function, but often results in fracture of the shell material owing to the enormous force that pronation at the sub-talar joint puts upon it.

The desired effect is for the orthosis to rock in the shoe. If the orthosis is required to rock, then it is made more functional by removing the medial anterior corner of the heel post. A point 1 cm proximal to the anterior border on the medial side is marked and a line is drawn at an angle of 45 degrees to the edge of the post. The material in this

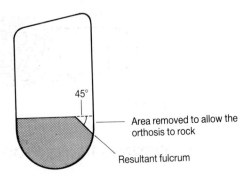

45°

Area removed to allow the
orthosis to rock

Resultant fulcrum

Fig. 7.28

area is removed, producing an edge which acts as a fulcrum and allows the orthosis to rock (Fig. 7.28).

There is one other very important technical detail to observe when
applying fore-foot posts, regardless of whether the post is for a varus
or valgus fore-foot anomaly. If the degree of correction is more than 3
degrees, the post must be extended to the most distal end of the toes.
Failure to do this will not only bring about a severe lip to the anterior
edge of the orthosis which will cause discomfort, but, more importantly,
in varus anomalies hallux flexus and ultimately hallux rigidus will
develop. This is due to the need for the hallux to plantar-flex to stabilise
the fore-foot at mid-stance (Fig. 7.29).

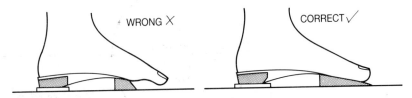

WRONG ✗   CORRECT ✓

Fig. 7.29

APPLICATION OF FORE-FOOT POST

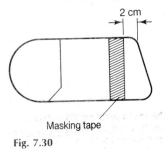

2 cm

Masking tape

Fig. 7.30

The fore-foot post extends on the lateral side of the shell from a point
2 cm proximal to the anterior border of the orthosis to the anterior border or beyond, depending on the degree of correction required. It
runs perpendicular to the long axis of the heel, and is therefore parallel to the anterior border of the heel post (Fig. 7.30).

Once the EVA material has been chosen, the preparation of the shell
and the method of application of the post is the same as for the heel
post.

It should be noted, however, that if the fore-foot post is to be extended to support the plantar surface of the fore-foot as well, it should
be extended also medially and laterally to reach the border of the
weight-bearing surface of the foot on both sides. This is essential to
prevent a ridge being felt in these areas (Fig. 7.31).

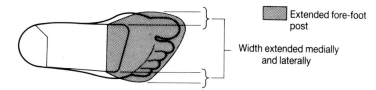

Fig. 7.31

GRINDING THE FORE-FOOT POST

The shell of the orthosis should still be firmly attached to the positive cast.

The most practical way to grind the fore-foot post is to hold the shell and cast so that the eyes of the operator are directly above the rear-foot post. The plantar surface of the previously ground rear-foot post is used as a guide. It should be positioned so that its longitudinal surface is parallel to an imaginary line running perpendicular to a transverse line positioned approximately 10 degrees below the centre of the working surface of the grinding wheel (Fig. 7.32 A and B). This allows a clear view of the work to be had by the operator.

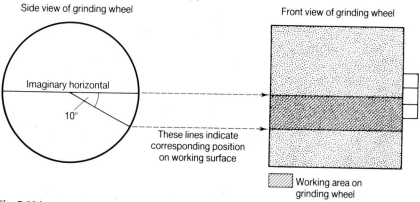

Fig. 7.32A

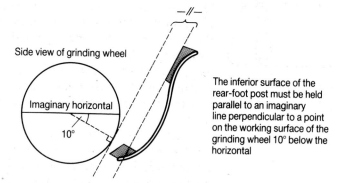

Fig. 7.32B

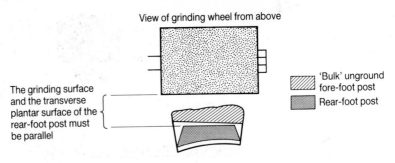

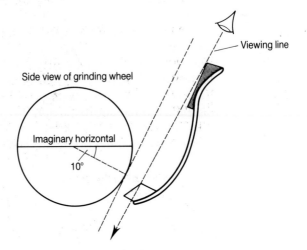

At this time the plantar surface of the rear-foot post should also be parallel transversely to the surface of the grinding wheel (Fig. 7.33).

This position is maintained very carefully as the operator looks down upon the proximal margin of the rear-foot post assimilating the position of the orthosis with regard to the grinding surface (Fig. 7.34).

Still with this position held firmly, the fore-foot post is presented to the grinder at the point 10 degrees below the horizontal and moved up and down slowly and in a line corresponding to the imaginary parallel lines already conceived (Fig. 7.35).

Grinding continues until the inferior anterior border of the shell of the orthosis comes into contact at its lowest point with the abrasive surface of the grinding wheel (Fig. 7.36).

The lowest point of the inferior anterior surface of the shell will be governed by the type of frontal plane anomaly which is being treated. If a varus post is being machined, the lowest point will be just lateral to the shaft of the fourth metatarsal. The valgus post will create a low point just underneath the shaft of the first metatarsal. Both of these low points will, of course, be on the anterior border of the shell (Fig. 7.37).

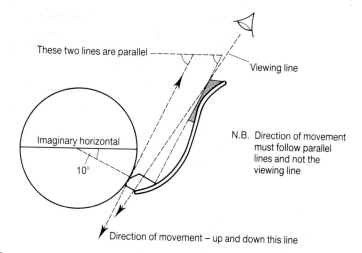

These two lines are parallel

Viewing line

Imaginary horizontal

10°

N.B. Direction of movement must follow parallel lines and not the viewing line

Direction of movement – up and down this line

Fig. 7.35

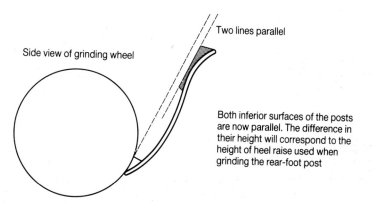

Side view of grinding wheel

Two lines parallel

Both inferior surfaces of the posts are now parallel. The difference in their height will correspond to the height of heel raise used when grinding the rear-foot post

Fig. 7.36

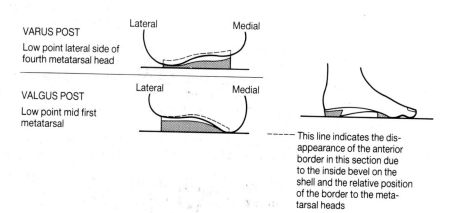

VARUS POST

Low point lateral side of fourth metatarsal head

Lateral   Medial

VALGUS POST

Low point mid first metatarsal

Lateral   Medial

------- This line indicates the disappearance of the anterior border in this section due to the inside bevel on the shell and the relative position of the border to the metatarsal heads

Fig. 7.37

The purpose of this particular grinding technique is to produce a correctly angled surface on the rear-foot and fore-foot posts so that both maintain firm ground contact longitudinally and transversely, when the heel is raised to the required height (Fig. 7.38).

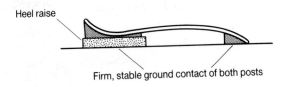

Fig. 7.38

Be sure to use the correct heel height when assessing the accuracy of this work.

If an error is made in the longitudinal angulation when grinding the fore-foot post, the post will not make ground contact along its proximal edge and a gap will be noticed between this edge and the supporting surface, when looking from the side (Fig. 7.39).

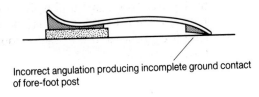

Fig. 7.39

Technically, this results in a pivot being formed by the anterior border of the shell and fore-foot post. This allows flexion and elongation of the shell, causing discomfort, fracture of the shell material and insufficient control of fore-foot function (Fig. 7.40).

Totally parallel surfaces on the rear and fore-foot posts are essential if the desired control is to be achieved.

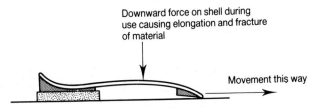

Fig. 7.40

AN ALTERNATIVE METHOD USED TO GRIND THE FORE-FOOT POST

When beginning the manufacture of functional foot orthoses, the method of parallel grinding that has been described may be difficult to grasp. There is another method that can be used which will result in the correct angulation being achieved.

Method

The rear-foot post is ground as described and the fore-foot posting material stuck to the shell. A piece of material of the thickness of the heel raise required is cut to roughly the same dimensions as the heel post and fixed to its plantar surface with some adhesive tape (Fig. 7.41).

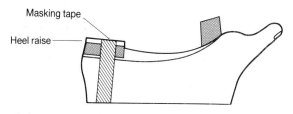

Masking tape

Heel raise

Fig. 7.41

All that is then required of the operator is to look straight down the plantar surface of this heightened rear-foot post when grinding. The orthosis is positioned on the grinding wheel as before and the fore-foot post is ground until it corresponds exactly in height to that of the rear-foot post. This can be checked by placing the orthosis on a flat surface, with the heel lift still stuck on with tape. Both the rear-foot and fore-foot posts should reach ground contact, both longitudinally and transversely (Fig. 7.42).

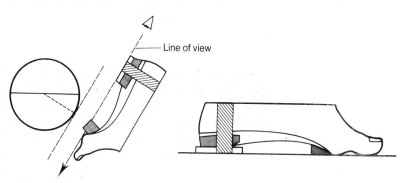

Line of view

Fig. 7.42

Once the correct relationship has been achieved, the heel raise can be removed. If done correctly, this method will achieve the desired result (Fig. 7.43).

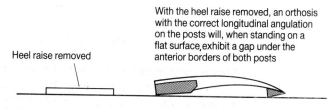

With the heel raise removed, an orthosis with the correct longitudinal angulation on the posts will, when standing on a flat surface, exhibit a gap under the anterior borders of both posts

Heel raise removed

Fig. 7.43

Either of these methods of grinding will produce a firm 'balanced' orthosis. However, if a 4 degree rock is required, a small amount of further grinding is necessary.

PRODUCTION OF THE ROCK TO ALLOW NORMAL PRONATION AT THE SUB-TALAR JOINT

This is achieved by grinding a small amount of posting material away from the medial side of the fore-foot post. With the shell still firmly attached to the positive cast and the rear-foot and fore-foot posts having been ground as described, the heel is raised to the required height and the work positioned on a flat surface. The tractograph is set by deducting 4 degrees from the rear-foot angle. It is then positioned so that its edge corresponds with the rear-foot bisection line. In order that the rear-foot bisection line corresponds with the tractograph setting, the cast and shell will require tipping medially (Fig. 7.44).

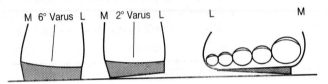

Fig. 7.44

A small amount of powered poster paint is spread on the table-top and the fore-foot post, once tipped medially, is rubbed lightly on the surface. This action will produce a mark on the medial inferior side of the fore-foot post indicating the point at which the grinding should be commenced.

A small amount is ground away from the marked area and the marking procedure repeated. Care must be taken in order to maintain the same criteria for grinding the fore-foot post as have already been described. This grinding and marking procedure is continued until the fore-foot post reaches full ground contact when the rear-foot post is raised to the required height and the cast tipped medially to represent 4 degrees of eversion of the calcaneus (Fig. 7.45). This will be indicated by the poster-paint marking the whole under surface of the fore-foot post.

Note

Although 4 degrees has been used in this example, the degree of sub-talar pronation that the clinician allows is governed by factors already discussed.

As has already been explained, this tipping is encouraged by producing a 45 degree grind-off on the medial anterior corner of the rear-foot

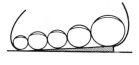

The purpose of the grind off is to leave the fore-foot post flat on the supporting surface when...

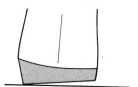

the rear-foot post is tilted sufficiently to allow a 4° reduction in the rear-foot angle
This allows the orthosis to rock during the heel lift phase of the gait cycle allowing normal sub-talar joint motion. It follows to assume that at heel strike and full-foot loading when the rear-foot post is firmly placed on the ground the fore-foot post will be lifted from the ground on the medial side

Fig. 7.45

post. The posting of the orthosis is now complete. The masking tape may be removed and a final polishing of the shell carried out, prior to the covering material of choice being applied.

COVERING THE ORTHOSIS

Covering an orthosis is relatively straightforward. However, the end result can be spoilt if a few small points are not observed.

Firstly, when applying contact adhesive to a covering that is going to extend further than the anterior border of the shell of the orthosis it pays to mark the position of the anterior border on the surface to be glued. This prevents glue being spread on an area that will not be adhered to, thus enhancing the professional appearance of the work (Fig. 7.46)

Secondly, when sticking the cover, it is wise to lay the glued cover gently on top of the orthosis. The cover is then pressed carefully downwards at the centre of the heel and the thumb is worked from the middle of the heel and up to the superior edge. From then onwards, work continues from the centre, spreading out towards the edges, thus expelling any trapped air in the process. When the heel seat is firmly stuck, adhesion of the cover can be completed by moving the hands distally. If air is trapped under the cover, a pin can be used to burst the bubbles although this is sometimes not very satisfactory.

Thirdly, the final trimming of the cover should be done with as much care as has been exercised on the manufacture. A razor-sharp knife is an ideal tool to use.

If adhesion is good and the cover is stuck right to the edges of the shell, the knife is simply run around the edges of the shell to remove the excess. The knife should be held perpendicularly to the superior edge of the shell. If preferred, scissors may be used to do this final trimming.

Covering material

Shell of orthosis

Spread no glue distal to the anterior border

Fig. 7.46

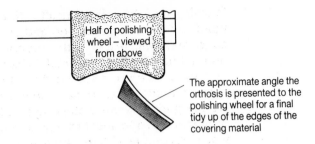

Half of polishing wheel – viewed from above

The approximate angle the orthosis is presented to the polishing wheel for a final tidy up of the edges of the covering material

Fig. 7.47

It is prudent, having completed the trimming, to use the polishing wheel to run around the edge of the orthosis. This tidies up any roughness and aids firm adhesion of the cover in this area (Fig. 7.47).

ACCOMMODATIVE FORE-FOOT EXTENSIONS

Frequently, lesions on the plantar surface of the fore-foot may require relief from the stresses of weight bearing. Hard corns and prominent metatarsophalangeal joints in the arthritic person are typical examples. The positive cast modifications that are necessary, and which I term

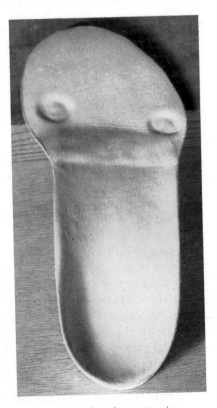

Plate 12 A full-length accommodative fore-foot extension.

'blowing out', have been dealt with in Chapter 5. If the necessary cast modifications are performed and an extended fore-foot post is used, concavities will result in the superior surface of this post when it is pressed to stick it to the shell. When grinding of the post takes place, care should be exercised not to reduce the thickness of the extended post too much, so as to maintain the effectiveness of those areas which are designed to relieve stress and redistribute pressure away from the prominences. On the first few attempts at this delicate procedure, I would recommend trial fitting with the patient prior to covering the orthosis. This will enable minor adjustments to be made in order to achieve the fine line between therapeutic advantage and the pad being too thick, which produces pressure on the dorsum of the fore-foot and toes, EVA is useful, but materials other than thermoplastic foams can be used for these extensions.

Note

It is necessary to increase the thickness of the heel post and the heel lift on an orthosis which has an accommodative fore-foot extension added. The reason becomes clear when consideration is given to the technical change that occurs to the longitudinal relationship of the fore-foot and rear-foot. If the fore-foot is raised by the necessary 3 or 4 mm, the accumulated effect is to raise the fore-foot in relationship to the rear-foot. This will make the heel of the wearer lower than the fore-foot, causing a slight dorsiflexion at the ankle joint. In a person with a limited range of motion at this joint, the wearing of such an orthosis would cause pain. The average person experiences mild discomfort and a small amount of aching in the calf muscles. Therefore, minimising this longitudinal difference is therapeutically advantageous and can be achieved by increasing the thickness of the rear-foot post as well as the thickness of the heel raise used when determining the heel height allowance of the orthosis.

The maximum possible increase in rear-foot post thickness is 5 mm, which includes the thickness of the shell. Greater thickness than this will lift the heel of the foot out of the heel seat of the shoe.

Technically, this process is achieved when grinding the rear-foot post by raising the anterior border of the shell of the orthosis the same amount as will be desired in the accommodative extension. Having done this, the heel raise allowance used when grinding the rear-foot post is also raised by the same amount. The rear-foot post is then ground in the manner that has been explained already, except in this situation the grinding of the post is complete when the rear-foot posting material is still 1–2 mm proud of the shell directly below the lowest part of the heel cup (Fig. 7.48).

This process raises the heel, maintains the parallel relationship of the inferior surfaces of both the rear-foot and fore-foot posts, producing the necessary control, as well as establishing the normal longitudinal relationship of the fore-foot and the rear-foot (Fig. 7.49).

If the normal heel raise method is used, a gap will form at the

Lowest part of heel cup

1–2 mm

Fig. 7.48

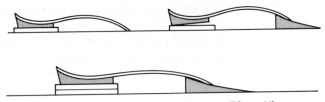

If the normal heel raise method is used, a gap will form at the anterior border of the rear-foot post. Simply altering the longitudinal angular grind to remove this gap will not increase the height of the rear-foot relative to the fore-foot. Therefore the thickness of the rear-foot post must also be increased as has been explained, so as to achieve the necessary results.

Fig. 7.49

proximal border of the rear-foot post. Simply altering the longitudinal angular grind to remove this gap will not increase the height of the rear-foot relative to the fore-foot. Therefore, the thickness of the rear-foot post must also be increased, as has been explained, so as to achieve the necessary results. See lower part of Figure 7.49.

It will be noted that the heel is raised by only 1–2 mm. While this is not necessarily the exact amount that the fore-foot has been raised by the accommodative extension, I am of the opinion that there is a certain amount of compression that occurs in the fore-foot posting material on weight bearing which minimises the height differential.

REAR-FOOT POSTING USING DENTAL ACRYLIC

Dental acrylic is invariably only used to obtain firm rear-foot control on orthoses. Its inflexibility means that it is most suited for use on rigid shell materials, otherwise the flexibility of the shell will cause the bond between the two to break and the acrylic to shear away during use. The decision on the rigidity of a shell material can be made using the weight to thickness ratio described earlier.

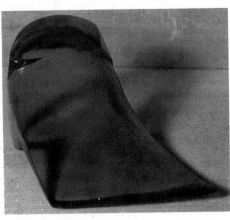

Plate 13 Dental acrylic used to post the rear-foot.

It could be contested by some that this method of gaining rear-foot control in an orthosis has been superseded by the development of very firm EVA. This is a matter for contention, but the method of using dental acrylic is described here in order to equip the reader with the complete armament of therapeutic possibilities.

Materials required

Cold cure monomer and polymer
Wet and dry sandpaper (120 grit)
Masking tape
EVA off-cuts
Polishing compound.

Tools/equipment

Wooden spatula
Small tinfoil dishes (type used for catering)
Cotton mop polishing wheel
A car tyre foot-pump—or compressed air on tap
A pressure pot (a vessel in which a pressure of 2 atmospheres can be reached).

Pressure pots are commercially available through dental suppliers. However, a converted pressure cooker is ideal. The tube in the centre of the lid which normally takes the weight is removed and replaced by a compressed air pipe attachment (Aro coupling). These are available from firms specialising in the manufacture or retail of air compressors. Depending on the make of pressure cooker, the hole in the lid may require enlarging to take this fitment. Some modern pressure cookers are not fitted with weights but simply have one pressure rating controlled by a spring-loaded valve which is activated when the pressure exceeds 2 atmospheres. With these models a separate hole must be drilled in the lid to take the compressed air pipe attachment. Once the fitting is in place, a suitable piece of tubing is assembled to connect the foot-pump to the pressure pot. To complete the home-made pressure vessel a little Vaseline is spread around the rubber seal inside the lid. This improves the efficiency of the seal.

Technique

1. The shell of the orthosis is manufactured and polished, and masking tape is applied to the anterior border of heel post area to prevent shell damage (Fig. 7.50).
2. The area to which the heel post is to be attached must now be prepared. Firstly, it is sanded using 120 grit paper, to roughen the area. Secondly, a series of shallow holes must be drilled 1 cm in from the perimeter of the heel of the orthosis. Six holes are sufficient, to a depth of half the thickness of the shell material. These holes act as a 'key' for the acrylic, preventing detachment (Fig. 7.51).

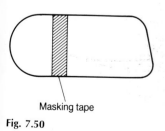

Masking tape

Fig. 7.50

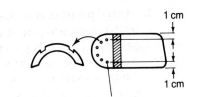

Roughened with sand paper

Fig. 7.51

3. A mould must now be made to hold the liquid acrylic while it is setting. The first step in producing the mould is to build up the anterior border of the heel post. An off-cut of 12 mm EVA is used. It is ground so that its proximal edge is totally flat. Contact adhesive is applied to the masking tape and to the EVA, and once dry and the EVA is at moulding temperature, the two are stuck together thus forming the anterior border of the heel post mould (Fig. 7.52).

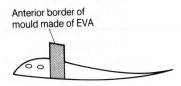

Anterior border of
mould made of EVA

Fig. 7.52

The medial and lateral edges of the EVA are ground to make them flush with the sides of the shell (Fig. 7.53).

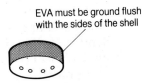

EVA must be ground flush
with the sides of the shell

Fig. 7.53 View of shell from posterior aspect of heel.

Masking tape is used to complete the mould, by sticking it to the medial edge of the EVA and then continuing it around the perimeter of the heel to attach it to the lateral side of the EVA (Fig. 7.54).

It is important that good adhesion is obtained with the masking tape all around the perimeter of the heel, otherwise leakage will occur when the acrylic is poured.

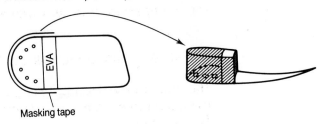

Masking tape

Fig. 7.54

4. At this point it is prudent to check that the shell sits relatively level in the pressure pot. If necessary, the shell should be propped up to prevent it tipping over. It is then removed and a little methyl methacrylate is painted over the surface of the heel area of the shell using a small brush similar to that found in a nail-varnish bottle. (A brush from a child's paint-box is an ideal substitute.) This process 'etches' the surface that is to have the acrylic applied to it, improving adhesion.

5. The pressure pot is now filled with tepid water to a level which will cover the shell and post of the orthosis.

   The cold cure acrylic can now be mixed. Thirty millilitres of the liquid monomer are drawn from the bottle; a syringe is suitable for the purpose. The monomer is put into a small tinfoil dish. Into the monomer is sprinkled the polymer powder. This is done slowly and the mixture is stirred all the time until a consistency of very runny cream is obtained. From this point, a working time of 1 minute is available. The acrylic should therefore be poured immediately into the heel post mould and the work transferred to the pressure pot. A skin is then allowed to form on the acrylic before the pressure is increased.

6. The lid is placed carefully on the pot so as not to disturb the work inside, and the pressure is increased to 2 atmospheres (2 kg/cm^2) using compressed air or the foot-pump. It is left undisturbed for 20 minutes.

7. When the time has been reached the pressure is released from the pot, the work removed and the mould taken off. The post is then ground in exactly the same way as has already been described for rear-foot posts.

8. Once grinding is complete, the sides of the acrylic are sanded by hand under cold running water using 180 grit wet and dry paper until *all* scratches have been removed. (It may also be smoothed using pumice powder, as was described for Rohadur.) The inferior surface of the post is best sanded by rubbing to and fro on a flat platform on which a piece of sandpaper is positioned.

When this process is satisfactorily completed, the acrylic is polished in the way already described for Rohadur.

Note

Dental acrylic can be cured without pressure but the end result is weak and full of holes. It is not worth attempting.

ALTERNATIVE MATERIAL FOR CONSTRUCTION OF MOULD

The mould in which the heel post is made can also be constructed using plasticine. (A method similar to this was first described by Mr J. T. Tillotson.)

Materials required

Plasticine
Rolling pin
Small sheet of glass with ground edges 80 × 80 mm.

Technique

Masking tape is applied to the shell distal to the anterior border of the heel post as before and the shell prepared in exactly the same way as has already been described, i.e. roughening with sandpaper and drilling six anchor holes. The masking tape is then removed and replaced just proximal to the anterior border of the heel post.

A strip of plasticine is rolled out so that it is long enough to span the width of the shell, i.e. 20 mm wide and 10 mm thick. This is applied across the width of the shell just distal to the anterior border of the heel post (Fig. 7.55).

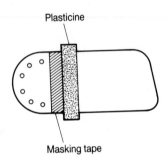

Fig. 7.55

The shell is then positioned on the positive cast and the rear-foot angle is set on the tractograph. The shell and the cast are positioned the right way up on a lightly dusted surface and positioned so that the line representing the rear-foot bisection corresponds to the angle set on the tractograph. The cast is now pressed firmly down on the supporting surface in order to squeeze the plasticine to the posting angle required. Remember to use the necessary heel raise when doing this and to take care to establish the correct posting angle.

The cast and shell are removed and any plasticine that has been squeezed proximally onto the masking tape is removed with a sharp knife, to produce a smooth straight edge. Furthermore, the medial and lateral edges are straightened up in the same way. The masking tape is then removed (Fig. 7.56).

The mould is completed by rolling out a further strip of plasticine of similar dimensions to the previous one but long enough to reach around the perimeter of the heel. It is attached on the medial side with its superior surface corresponding exactly to the superior surface of the strip representing the anterior border of the mould at this point.

It is placed carefully around the heel and is attached on the lateral

Cut away excess plasticine
along distal edge of masking
tape and then remove tape

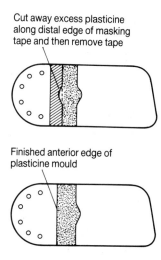

Finished anterior edge of
plasticine mould

Fig. 7.56

Anterior edge of mould

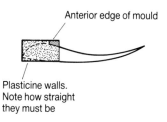

Plasticine walls.
Note how straight
they must be

Fig. 7.57

Glass

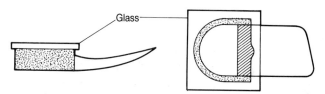

Fig. 7.58

side at the same height as the superior surface of the anterior border of the mould at this point.

Care must be exercised to keep these walls of the mould straight (Fig. 7.57).

Good adhesion must be achieved at all junctions of this mould. With the mould completed, methyl methacrylate is used to etch the surface of the shell onto which the acrylic is to be poured. The acrylic is mixed and poured carefully into the mould until it reaches the top all round. The piece of glass is then gently pressed on top of the mould. It adheres to the plasticine, so preventing leakage of the acrylic and establishing the inferior surface of the posting platform (Fig. 7.58). The prepared work is then put into the pressure pot as before and allowed to set under pressure.

When the work is removed from the pressure pot, the plasticine is removed and any grinding necessary to tidy up the work is done as described previously.

There is little to chose between the two methods except that the second method requires slightly less work on the grinder to complete.

General

Undoubtedly much practice will follow the reading of this chapter before sufficient skill is acquired to gain proficiency.

However, if the basic principles that have been described are followed, a sound start will have been made which can be developed slowly.

The fundamental principles of cleanliness and forethought will avoid unnecessary mess which in all cases compromises the professional appearance of the finished article.

If thought is given at all times to the comfort of the foot of the wearer, then many technical mistakes will be avoided and you will enjoy your work all the more.

8

Ethylene vinyl acetate (EVA) orthoses

I have already stated my opinion on the virtues of ethylene vinyl acetate when used in podiatric applications. In this chapter I wish to describe the techniques involved in manufacturing functional and accommodative orthoses using this material. These orthoses were designed and developed by Mr J T Tillotson (of Wellington, New Zealand) and myself. They owe their conception to a personal drive towards improving the mobility of people suffering the cruelties of rheumatoid arthritis. They also represent an attempt to redress the therapeutic balance, which too often is becoming weighted in favour of the financially more secure.

It is my belief that the quality of life for people suffering from rheumatoid arthritis is often reduced by the severity of the pain in their feet, as the mobility so necessary for an independent lifestyle and optimal systemic health is restricted. We are still ignorant of the causative agents, exact aetiology and cures of this and many other arthritides. However, if we can reduce the pain and improve mobility for these people we can return in part something they have lost.

Experimentation began using polyurethane foam. (We are grateful for the assistance of Mr Ron Cribb of VITA (NZ) in this work.) However, polyurethane foams did not altogether suit our purpose and the isocyanate materials used in their manufacture have their own inherent dangers. Ethylene vinyl acetate became the material of choice and led to the development of the orthosis. The development and clinical trials were spread over five years and have resulted in a therapeutic aid which reaches beyond our initial hopes and expectations. Not only are these orthoses suitable for patients suffering from systemic arthritis, but also for the elderly for whom osteo-arthrosis has limited the ranges of joint motion in their feet. This makes control and shock absorption all the more essential.

These orthoses are cushioning and can redistribute pressure from, and cushion, lesions. They also control the function of the foot. Combining these properties appears to reduce inflammation in the joints of the lower limb. Consequently, when used in arthritis in conjunction with skilful medical therapies, judiciously prescribed EVA orthoses may help to slow the rate of deterioration of the articular facets. (The predilection the different arthritides have for different joints should always be borne in mind so that the most beneficial therapy is achieved.)

These orthoses have also shown themselves to be of value in maintaining the integrity of the insensitive foot in diabetes and in other conditions which can result in pedal insensitivity. Their properties also make them ideally suited for children's orthoses. Furthermore, the frequent renewals necessary with growth do not over-stretch the financial capabilities of parents. They do however require skilful adaptation if they are to be used to treat the hypermobile foot which requires more rigid control. (A suitable method of adaptation will be given later.)

The range of uses of this material is gauged by its density; this is related to the weight of the patient and the function required. Its use in general terms is limited only by the imagination of the practitioner. EVA machines well, and with a few hours' practice, a fine, aesthetically pleasing orthosis can be produced within little more than 10 minutes machine time. Therefore EVA enables the manufacture of unique and economic forms of functional and accommodative orthoses. These have the potential of providing relief for many patients.

THE ALL-IN-ONE ORTHOSIS

This type of orthosis is so named because it is an integral unit. The shell, posts and fore-foot accommodative extension are moulded and then machined in one operation. The name is in itself unimportant. For the purpose of this text it serves as an indication of the mode of manufacture and the inherent reduction in handling time required to produce these orthoses.

However, while being quick to make, a high degree of skill, both technical and empathic, is required to grind these orthoses successfully. To avoid disappointment, I would recommend mastery of the basic grinding skills mentioned earlier, before the manufacture of these orthoses is attempted.

CONSTRUCTION TECHNIQUES

The positive casts on which these orthoses are moulded are produced and modified in exactly the same way as has already been described. There are three basic methods of using EVA as a means of constructing a functional/accommodative foot orthosis:

1. The moulding and grinding of a shell and post in one operation without an allowance for an accommodative fore-foot extension. This orthosis looks much like a rigid or semi-flexible orthosis. However, the clinician is able to gain control of the foot while allowing greater cushioning and shock absorption where necessary. Mastery of this technique is fundamental to EVA orthosis construction.

2. The moulding and grinding of a shell, post and accommodative extension all in one operation. The blending of more than one density of EVA is possible prior to moulding, if different qualities are required of different areas of the orthosis. The technique is an expansion of Technique 1.
3. The moulding and grinding of a shell and post in one operation with the fore-foot extension added secondarily. This is the best method when additional materials with qualities not found in EVA are required.

Many therapeutic variations may be adopted once these fundamental techniques have been mastered. The scope is restricted, as mentioned previously, only by the imagination of the practitioner. Some permutations which I have found useful will be explained later in the text.

Materials required

EVA of differing densities, depending on the weight of the patient and the therapeutic requirements (see Table 8.1)

Table 8.1 Patient's weight : EVA density ratios. The weight/density relating to the shells and posts will produce control within the joints of the foot. To initiate greater shock absorption, the density of the material is reduced for any given weight. It is also possible to 'fine-tune' these ratios by knowing the exact weight of the patient. The density given for the accommodation extension will provide redistribution of pressure; reduce the density for more shock absorption

Patient's weight	Ethylene vinyl acetate (Measured in density of foam) (kg/m^3)	
	Shells and Posts	Accommodative extensions
Less than 25 kg	220	75–85
More than 25 kg but Less than 45 kg	240	75–85
More than 45 kg but Less than 75 kg	260	140–180
More than 75 kg	300–360	220

Contact adhesive
Vinyl covering material
Chinagraph pencil.

Tools and equipment

A razor-sharp knife
Band saw
Scissors
Oven
A press.

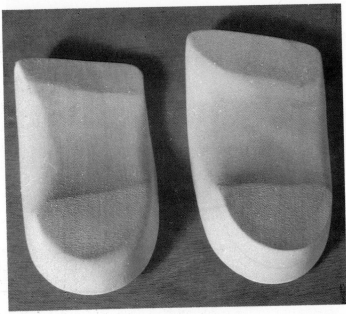

Plate 14 The underside of the EVA orthosis, showing the integral nature of the shell and post. This can be achieved using one sheet of EVA, if the convex dome of the plantar surface of the heel is not great (left). If the amount of doming requires it, two pieces of EVA must be joined in the area of the heel, to enable to flat platform of sufficient width to be created in this area (right).

Technique I (The moulding of a shell and post in one operation)

Manufacturing steps:

1. The EVA is chosen in the density required. It must be 12 mm thick. It is cut to the standard blank dimension of 10 cm × 20 cm, either with a razor-sharp knife or on a band-saw.
2. The amount of material used per orthosis depends largely on the height of the longitudinal arch and the degree of convexity of the plantar surface of the heel. A foot with a high arch or a particularly domed heel will require two sheets of 12 mm to be stuck together, while a foot of average dimensions will require only one sheet. If two sheets are to be joined, they must not be joined until the first sheet has been moulded to the positive cast. Any attempt to mould 24 mm in one operation is too demanding for most presses and results in an imperfectly shaped orthosis.
3. The lines drawn on the positive cast during the marking-out procedure are now reinforced using a chinagraph pencil. This will aid manufacture, as will be seen.
4. The material is heated in an oven until mouldable (3–5 minutes), and is then pressed onto the positive cast in exactly the same way described for semi-flexible and rigid materials. It is preferable to allow the material to cool completely before removing it from the press. However, if this is not feasible the material can be removed from the press after 5 minutes and then bandaged to the positive

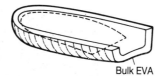

Bulk EVA

- - - - - Line denoting the borders
of the orthosis. This line
was transferred from the
positive cast during
moulding, having been
reinforced with a
chinagraph pencil.

Fig. 8.1

cast until it has thoroughly cooled. This will ensure a perfect moulding.

5. The orthosis may now be shaped and ground.
6. It will be noticed that the chinagraph pencil markings, having been subjected to heat, have melted and been transferred faithfully to the inside surface of the moulded EVA (Fig. 8.1) This transfer of markings allows accurate 'gross' removal of the waste material to be performed on a band-saw. (Please review the text relating to the use of this tool before beginning this procedure (pp. 72 and 73.)
7. When the gross waste material has been removed, the basic shape of the orthosis will be apparent. The accuracy of the anterior border of the orthosis must be checked and tidied up on the grinding wheel.
8. The inferior surface of the orthosis, which will be in contact with the insole of the shoe, is now ground to match the rear-foot frontal plane measurement established in the clinical examination. This means that, unlike the posts on the semi-flexible and rigid orthoses, the *whole* of the under surface of the EVA is at this stage ground to this measurement. The pronatory allowance at the fore-foot is ground secondarily. The method of achieving this angle has been

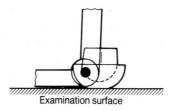

Examination surface

The rear-foot bisection line is angled
to correspond to the frontal plane
measurement established by
clinical examination. With the
tractograph set, the cast and shell
are rubbed to and fro longitudinally.
<u>No</u> heel raise is used when marking.

Fig. 8.2 Marking the inferior surface of the EVA on a dusted surface.

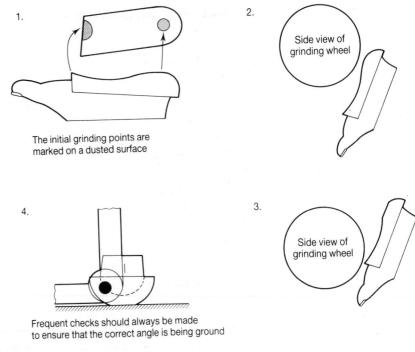

1.

The initial grinding points are marked on a dusted surface

2.

Side view of grinding wheel

3.

Side view of grinding wheel

4.

Frequent checks should always be made to ensure that the correct angle is being ground

Fig. 8.3

described. The method of transferring it to the material using a tractograph and a surface lightly dusted with poster paint is identical to that described earlier in the heel posting technique, except for one variation, no heel raise is necessary when marking the posts on the EVA orthosis (Fig. 8.2).

9. Having marked the underside of the EVA on a flat surface (with no heel raise), the material, still positioned on the cast, is presented to the grinding wheel 10 degrees below the horizontal. The centre of the mark made on the heel is presented first and a small amount of EVA is ground away. The centre of the mark made under the anterior border is then presented and a similar amount is ground away there. At this point the accuracy of the frontal plane angulation is checked before proceeding further (Fig. 8.3).

10. The grinding is continued until the EVA is reduced to 1 mm in thickness at its lowest point on the anterior border (i.e. this will be just laterally to the fourth metatarsophalangeal joint in varus deformities, and under the first metatarsophalangeal joint in valgus deformities). At this time the surface under the lowest point of the heel should also be 1 mm in thickness. This means that a flat grind has been achieved along the whole length of the orthosis. Be sure to check the depth of the material frequently during the grinding process, so as not to 'go through' in any area. Great sensitivity will be developed in the thumb and index finger when used as callipers to establish the depth (Fig. 8.4).

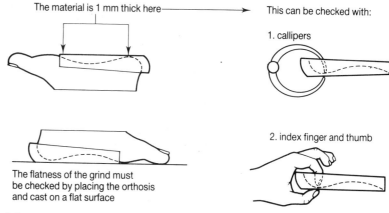

Fig. 8.4

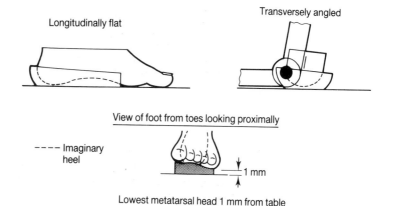

Fig. 8.5

The accuracy of the transfer of the correct frontal plane measurement should be frequently checked also during the grinding procedure. The result of this grind will be a longitudinally flat, yet transversely angled inferior surface to the EVA. The lowest metatarsal head should be 1 mm above the examination surface when viewed from the side (Fig. 8.5).

Note If a heel raise is required for any reason, the anterior border is still ground until it is 1 mm in thickness. However, the thickness of the material under the heel is only reduced until the heel height that is required has been achieved. This can be measured with a pair of callipers (Fig. 8.6).

11. The next step is to shape accurately the superior surface of the sides and heel seat of the orthosis, the bulk having already been removed on the band-saw. If a band-saw is unavailable, the total bulk can be removed on the grinding wheel. The superior surfaces of all sides are ground by presenting them to the grinding wheel, the heel facing down towards the floor and the under surface,

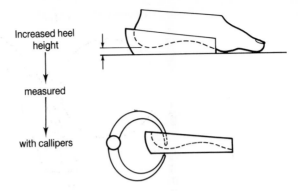

Increased heel height

↓

measured

↓

with callipers

Fig. 8.6

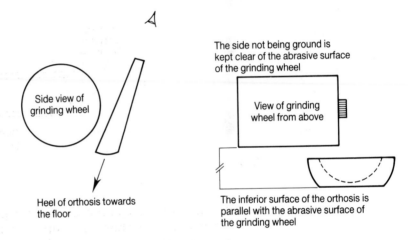

Side view of grinding wheel

Heel of orthosis towards the floor

The side not being ground is kept clear of the abrasive surface of the grinding wheel

View of grinding wheel from above

The inferior surface of the orthosis is parallel with the abrasive surface of the grinding wheel

Fig. 8.7

which has already been ground to frontal plane angle required, facing the operator and *parallel* to the grinding surface of the wheel. The medial and lateral sides are ground independently.

When working on an orthosis for the left foot the medial side is ground on the right-hand side of the wheel, while the lateral side is ground on the left. This process is reversed when working on an orthosis for the right foot. This keeps the side that is not being ground away from the abrasive surface, reducing the risk of mistakes (Fig. 8.7).

The aim is to tidy up the superior surface and shape it accurately to the markings made by the chinagraph pencil during pressing. Great care must be taken so as not to 'grind out' the medial arch, particularly as the arch area is being ground in a way I discouraged you from practising when making the semi-flexible and rigid orthoses. The method described here is necessary when working EVA owing to the flexibility of the material. This allows it to oscillate if worked in the same way as other materials. The border will not be 'ground out' if a longitudinal rocking motion is exercised while grinding (Fig. 8.8).

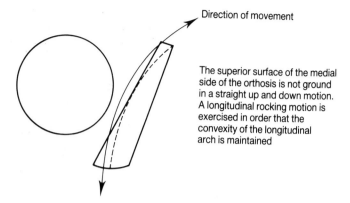

Direction of movement

The superior surface of the medial side of the orthosis is not ground in a straight up and down motion. A longitudinal rocking motion is exercised in order that the convexity of the longitudinal arch is maintained

Fig. 8.8

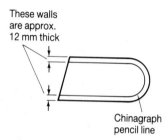

These walls are approx. 12 mm thick

Chinagraph pencil line

Fig. 8.9

12. When the tidying up procedure is complete it will be noticed that the sides of the orthosis are approximately 12 mm thick, depending on the amount of EVA used (Fig. 8.9). These sides must now be reduced in thickness, to no less than 3 mm.

This is achieved by presenting the side of the orthosis to the grinding wheel, with the heel facing the ground once again. The reduction is started at the anterior end of the orthosis and run down the side and around the heel to its mid-point. The same is then done with the other side of the orthosis until the mid-point of the heel is reached again. While grinding, a slight taper is put on the sides so as to allow a snug fit within the shoe (Fig. 8.10).

It is important, at this point, to envisage carefully the shape of the insole of the shoe into which the orthosis is to be placed. Shoes are not straight longitudinally, they are invariably inflared to some degree (Fig. 8.11.) This means that the inferior surface of the orthosis must also be inflared to the same degree, otherwise a significant bulge will result on the medial side of the 'upper' of the shoe. The inflare is ground by increasing the angle of the taper in the area of the medial arch. The best way to develop this skill is to practise by making a template of the insole of the shoe into which the orthosis is to be placed. Trace around this on the under surface of the EVA, which has been ground to the frontal plane angle required. Practise developing the insole shape, while main-

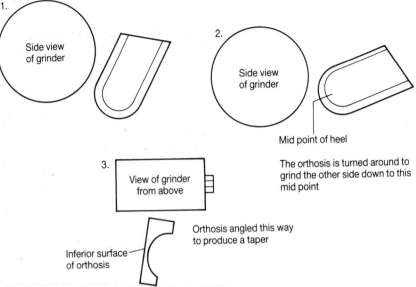

Fig. 8.10

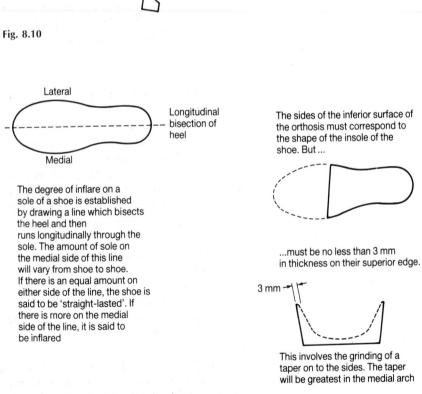

Fig. 8.11 Inflare in the sole of a shoe.

taining the correct dimensions of the orthosis and the superior borders to no less than 3 mm thick.

(This is best learnt on an orthosis for your own shoe for which you can easily fashion a template.)

> **Note**
>
> I mention here practising using a template of your own shoe. I have found it invaluable to have a modified positive cast of my own feet available at all times. It enables experimentation and teaches subtly of technique in the search for comfort.

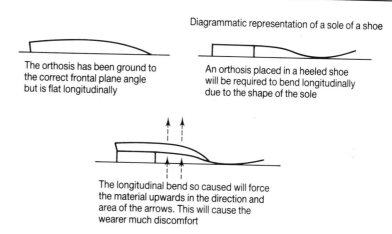

Diagrammatic representation of a sole of a shoe

The orthosis has been ground to the correct frontal plane angle but is flat longitudinally

An orthosis placed in a heeled shoe will be required to bend longitudinally due to the shape of the sole

The longitudinal bend so caused will force the material upwards in the direction and area of the arrows. This will cause the wearer much discomfort

Fig. 8.12

13. The orthosis as it stands has the functional correction (the posting) ground on its inferior surface, and the sides tapered. It will not yet be functional because it is flat on its under surface, and when put into a shoe with a heel will be required to bend longitudinally. The next and important step is to grind away some material from the under surface to allow it to bend in the shoe. If this is not done, it will indeed bend under body weight, but in doing so, will push up the medial arch causing the wearer discomfort (Fig. 8.12).

   In order to grind away the correct amount of material to allow the orthosis to bend, two lines are first drawn. One line is drawn across the underside of the orthosis to correspond to the distal margin of the rear-foot post and one to represent the proximal margin of the fore-foot post (Fig. 8.13).

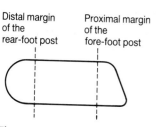

Distal margin of the rear-foot post   Proximal margin of the fore-foot post

Fig. 8.13 View of the underside of the orthosis.

   Some of the material between these two lines is then ground away to produce an arch shape. This prevents the bend in the shoe, created by the raised heel, from pushing the arch of the orthosis upwards.

   The under surface of the orthosis is presented to the grinding wheel and slid to and fro sideways to remove some material. It is angled slightly towards the medial side so that a little more material is removed medially than is removed laterally. This operation is best carried out with the heel of the orthosis facing uppermost (Fig. 8.14).

   The work is continued until, when viewed from the side, the two lines drawn are connected by a neat arch (Fig. 8.15).

14. At this stage, if a varus posting position of the fore-foot was achieved

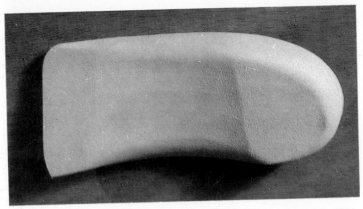

Plate 15 The arch shape that must be ground into the under surface of the EVA orthosis.

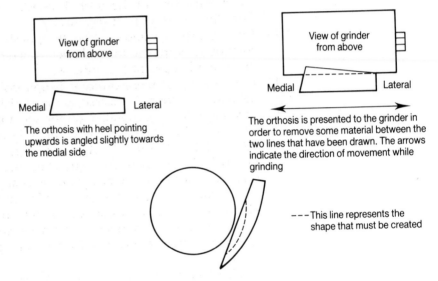

View of grinder from above

Medial · Lateral

The orthosis with heel pointing upwards is angled slightly towards the medial side

View of grinder from above

Medial · Lateral

The orthosis is presented to the grinder in order to remove some material between the two lines that have been drawn. The arrows indicate the direction of movement while grinding

– – –This line represents the shape that must be created

Fig. 8.14

Side view of the orthosis

The arch formed by the removal of material between the lines drawn, enables the orthosis to bend longitudinally in a heeled shoe without the material in the area of the arch being forced upwards

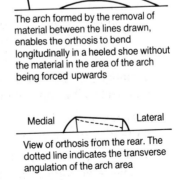

Medial · Lateral

View of orthosis from the rear. The dotted line indicates the transverse angulation of the arch area

Fig. 8.15

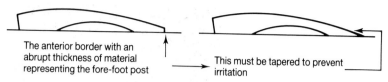

The anterior border with an abrupt thickness of material representing the fore-foot post

This must be tapered to prevent irritation

Fig. 8.16

when the initial posting was ground as in Steps 8 and 9 and which is sufficient to require a reduction to allow pronation at the subtalar joint, the necessary amount is now removed from the fore-foot post. This is done in the way already described for the procedure when making the rigid and semi-flexible orthoses.

15. Once the fore-foot posting angulation is complete the superior surface of the anterior border must be ground to reduce the bulk on the highest side of the post. This will avoid the risk of irritation from the fore-foot post (Fig. 8.16).

16. The orthosis is completed on the polishing wheel. No polishing compound is applied to the wheel, which is used simply to smooth the ground edges of the orthosis.

17. The covering of these orthoses is optional as functionally it is not needed. If a cover is desired, the material of choice is vinyl, with or without foam, depending on the therapeutic requirements. The vinyl must be heated for 30 seconds in an oven set at between 160° and 170° Celsius. Heating for longer than this will melt the material. The vinyl is then stretched over the positive cast and stapled in position. Contact adhesive is applied to it and to the inside surface of the orthosis; it is allowed to become 'touch' dry. The orthosis is then positioned carefully on the vinyl and pressed firmly. The staples are removed from the vinyl, the covered orthosis is removed from the cast and the covering material trimmed with scissors.

It is important that the covering of these orthoses is done in this way. If an attempt is made to simply apply the covering material to the orthosis without first heating it and stretching it over the cast, the elasticity in it will pucker the relatively flexible walls of the orthosis, thus disfiguring them.

18. The orthosis is now ready for issue. The actual time taken in manufacture is unlikely to be more than 10 to 15 minutes, depending on whether a cover has been added.

Technique II (The moulding of a shell, post and accommodative extension all in one operation)

This technique is an extension of Technique I and is valuable in two particular instances:

- When the degree of fore-foot posting of the foot at mid-stance is severe enough to lift the fore-foot, at the anterior border of the orthosis, *more than* 3 mm from the supporting surface

- When prominent, painful weight-bearing areas of the foot distal to the anterior border of the orthosis require cushioning or pressure to be redistributed away from them (sometimes both).

Some general points

1. The thickness of shell material required for the orthosis depends largely, as before, on the height of the longitudinal arch and the shape of the heel. The same criteria are used as were described in Technique 1, Step 2.
2. If the fore-foot extension to be moulded is required to redistribute pressure away from painful areas of the plantar surface of the fore-foot, the cast must be modified correctly. The plaster enlargement of the lesions, is carried out as was described in the 'blowing-out' procedure.
3. The length of the piece of material used for these orthoses depends on the foot size and the length of the extension required; it is advisable to measure each cast.
4. The EVA material must be chosen in the density required. Three things govern this choice:

   a. The control/shock-absorption required in the shell.
   b. The redistributive properties required in the fore-foot extension.
   d. The cushioning properties required in the fore-foot extension (and perhaps in the shell as well).

Blending of any number of densities of EVA can be achieved prior to moulding. However, if the blending involves increasing the thickness of EVA above 12 mm, do remember to press the layers individually, one on top of the other, to ensure perfect moulding. Each layer must be allowed to cool before another is attached.

However, if a therapeutic advantage is thought to be gained by adding a lining of open- or closed-cell foam rubber sheeting to the EVA, the rubber may be glued to the EVA *prior* to heating and moulding. This ensures that the rubber, when moulded inside the EVA, not only keeps its shape, but does not reduce the amount of room within the orthosis, as it would had it been added after the moulding of the shell. This latter consideration is important when using lining rubbers of thicknesses *greater* than 3 mm.

Methods of blending densities of EVA with other materials are shown in Figures 8.17 A and B.

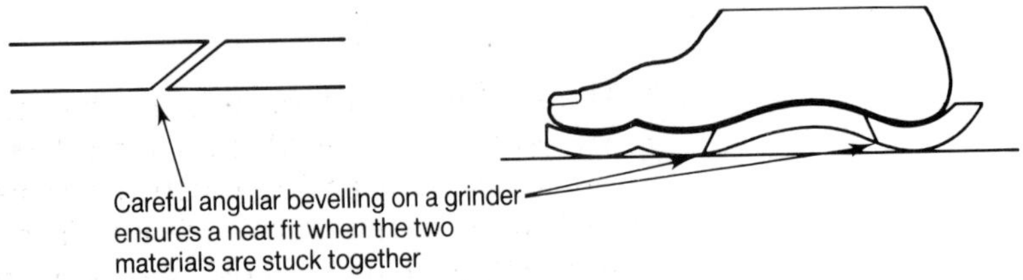

Careful angular bevelling on a grinder ensures a neat fit when the two materials are stuck together

Fig. 8.17A Longitudinal blending.

The foot is on this side

	Soft EVA
	Hard EVA

This combination when moulded and ground will achieve firm control from the hard under-layer of EVA, while still allowing shock absorption by way of the absorbent inner layer. The combination of materials would be moulded in *two* operations.

	Plastazote or soft polyethylene foam
	Rubber foam
	EVA

This combination could offer control with much cushioning, particularly for the arthritic. A combination of materials such as this with just one layer of EVA, would be moulded in one operation, the layers having been stuck together prior to moulding.

Fig. 8.17B Building layers.

In many instances, where fore-foot extensions are required simply because of the height of posting, no blending of materials is needed. In all instances where fore-foot extensions are required, moulding materials in one or more operations prior to grinding produces perfectly contoured orthoses of superior quality and comfort. The technique is worth mastering.

Manufacturing steps

1. The lines drawn on the cast during the marking-out procedure are reinforced using a chinagraph pencil. The medial and lateral borders of the fore-foot should also be drawn in (Fig. 8.18).

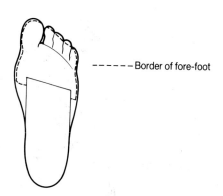

- - - - - Border of fore-foot

Fig. 8.18

2. The heating of the material is identical to step 4, Technique I.
3. The gross removal of the excess EVA is now done on the bandsaw or grinder and is much the same as in Technique I, except that the excess is removed only from around the heel and down the length of the orthosis to 1 cm proximal to the first and fifth metatarsal heads (Fig. 8.19).

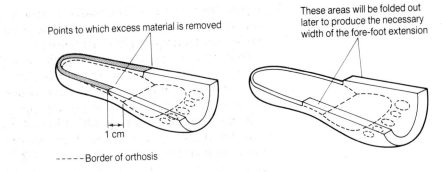

Points to which excess material is removed

These areas will be folded out later to produce the necessary width of the fore-foot extension

1 cm

- - - - - Border of orthosis

Fig. 8.19

4. The anterior border of the orthosis will not of course be cut, now that the fore-foot extension is integral. It will, nevertheless, be evident on the inside, from the chinagraph pencil marking. It is important to know exactly where it is, so that the fore-foot posting that will be ground into the orthosis is positioned correctly and the area of the anterior border reduced to the necessary thickness. Once experience is gained, you will undoubtedly develop a 'feel' for establishing the border. However, I would recommend that when initially attempting this technique, two pins are pushed through the EVA from the inside. One pin is positioned on the medial side of the anterior border and one on the lateral side. A mark is made at the points where they emerge on the underside of the orthosis, and the points are joined by a line which is extended to the medial and lateral sides of the orthosis. This then transfers the anterior border to the underside of the orthosis and denotes the area on to which to concentrate in the initial grind (Fig. 8.20).

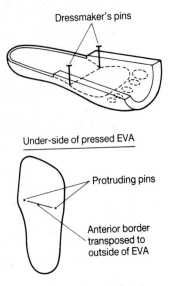

Dressmaker's pins

Under-side of pressed EVA

Protruding pins

Anterior border transposed to outside of EVA

Fig. 8.20

5. If you have practised Technique I, you will now be able to mark out and grind the correct frontal plane angulation into the orthosis, while maintaining longitudinal flatness.

This now is carried out using the anterior border line as the anterior marker. You can ignore the fore-foot extension just for this moment. However, as the grind proceeds, one thought must govern your actions, i.e. the purpose of the extension.

If the extension is being added in order to negate the problems associated with large degrees of fore-foot posting, the anterior *border is reduced to 1 mm in thickness at its lowest point*. This is just as has been done in Technique I, and as such includes the same thickness at the rear-foot. Furthermore, the thickest part of the extension should not be greater than 5 mm (Fig. 8.21).

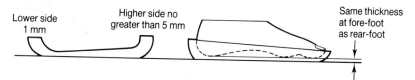

Fig. 8.21

However, if the extension is being added to provide shock absorption, and there is a frontal plane anomaly at the fore-foot, then the anterior border is reduced until 3 mm of thickness remains *at its lowest point*. This is very important and an essential step in the manufacture of these devices. If more than this amount of material is left, the foot will be raised in the shoe and may become rubbed, particularly on the dorsum of the toes. If less than this, when the weight to density ratio given is followed, insufficient shock absorption will be achieved. Lastly, if the extension is being added to provide redistribution to prominent plantar lesions, then the grind at this stage should leave not less than 4 mm at the anterior border and rear-foot.

(Remember, this depth corresponds to the average depth of cast addition when 'blowing-out' (Fig. 8.22).)

6. Once the frontal plane angulation of the shell is complete, the angulation may be ground into the fore-foot extension, which (in a sagittal and transverse section) will be noticed at this stage to be bending upwards slightly (Fig. 8.23).

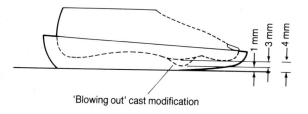

'Blowing out' cast modification

Fig. 8.22

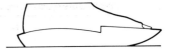

Fig. 8.23

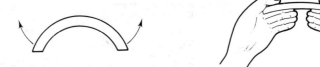

Fig. 8.24

This bend must be straightened to present the extension to the grinder. It is a bit like trying to turn a rather tough empty grapefruit skin half inside-out. The sides must be pulled up to establish some flatness (Fig. 8.24).

The under surface of the flattened extension is presented to the grinder and the frontal plane angulation is ground.

This grind follows the angulation established at the anterior border of the orthosis, which was the straight-through grind, from the rear-foot. Care must be taken when grinding the extensions that are added to redistribute pressure. The extension must be reduced slowly, using the index finger and thumb as callipers, so that dimples created by the 'blow outs' on the cast are not inadvertently ground in to. The grind ceases when a maximum of 1 mm of material underlies the dimple.

A measurement is now taken of the thickness of the material surrounding the dimples and the material under the anterior border and rear-foot post is reduced to a similar thickness (Fig. 8.25).

7. If the material extends to the distal end of the toes, the upper surface of the extension may now be ground to remove the mound of material created by the EVA sinking into the webbing space during moulding. There is often also a thickened ridge of material that bends around the sides and ends of the toes. These projec-

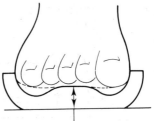

The thickness of the material surrounding the dimpled 'blow-out' modification is measured

Fig. 8.25

Sagittal cross section of orthosis

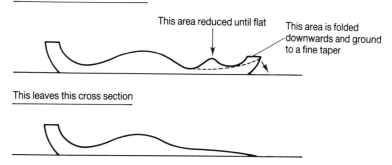

This area reduced until flat

This area is folded downwards and ground to a fine taper

This leaves this cross section

Fig. 8.26

tions are smoothed off on the grinder, and the extension is at the same time ground to a fine taper at the *distal* end. This prevents pressure on the nails. The medial and lateral sides are left at full thickness (Fig. 8.26).

Obviously, if special foams have been added to the inside of the orthosis at the moulding stage, the procedure just mentioned will remove parts of the foam. Therefore, if foam is added, remember two things:

a. Use plaster of Paris to fill the depression formed by the webbing space before moulding the materials and, at the same time level off any dorsal curvature of the toes to render the cast flat distal to the metatarsophalangeal joints. *This modification is done at the same time as the main modification* (Fig. 8.27).

b. The taper produced at the distal end of the extension is ground underneath. The material will 'bed down' in the shoe after a day or two of wear (Fig. 8.28).

Dorsal curvature of apex of toes 'squared off'

Depression formed by webbing space levelled off

} Use plaster of Paris

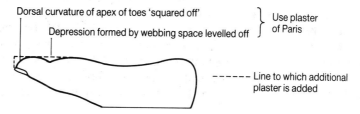

- - - - - Line to which additional plaster is added

Care must be taken to only add plaster distal to the metatarsophalangeal joints

Fig. 8.27

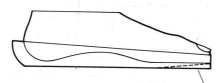

Taper ground underneath when this type of modification is used because foam is added at the stage of 'pressing'

Fig. 8.28

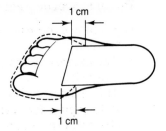

Fig. 8.29

8. The sides of the orthosis are shaped as described in Technique I. As always, as was emphasised in the manufacture of semi-flexible and rigid orthoses, when fore-foot extensions are added they must follow the line of the border of the foot from 1 cm proximal to the anterior border of the orthosis. They therefore widen at this point, a fact that must be remembered during grinding (Fig. 8.29).

9. Once the sides have been ground, the sides of the fore-foot extension are checked to establish their accuracy with the shape of the fore-foot.

10. The under surface of the orthosis must now be ground to allow it to bend in the shoe. Follow, Technique 1 step 13.

11. A cover may now be added, if desired, using the method described in Technique I, otherwise the orthosis is ready for issue.

Technique III (The moulding of a shell and post in one operation, with a fore-foot extension added secondarily)

This technique is valuable when materials that will not 'heat mould' yet have qualities not found in EVA are required for use in the fore-foot extension. The technique is a straightforward expansion of Technique I, which is followed in every detail and completed, except for covering, before the addition of the separate fore-foot extension.

The material used for the extension can be whatever is thought to be therapeutically advantageous. It can have holes cut in it, conventional padding incorporated in it, and be full length (to apex of the toes) or go only far as the webbing space.

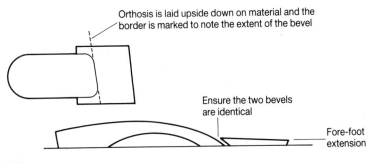

Orthosis is laid upside down on material and the border is marked to note the extent of the bevel

Ensure the two bevels are identical

Fore-foot extension

Fig. 8.30

The only specific requirements of the material are:

1. It follows the rule of increased width, as do all extended posts or covers.
2. The extension 'marries' exactly into the anterior border of the EVA orthosis.

   This is achieved by creating a 'bottom', or 'under-bevel', on the extension, identical in angulation to the 'top', or 'over-bevel', on the anterior border of the orthosis (Fig. 8.30).
3. Once the extension is stuck, the orthosis is covered to strengthen the joint between the two materials and prevent avulsion of the extension.

   Also, some rubbers cling to hose materials, causing slight discomfort and preventing the shoe from being put on easily. A suitable cover will overcome this.

9
Adaptations of the EVA orthoses

Adaptations of the techniques already described in Chapter 8 are beneficial when:

1. Heel pain is the primary symptom experienced
2. Increased control of the sub-talar joint is required
3. Control of the sub-talar joint is required but with extra cushioning, i.e. when treating the arthritic foot.

HEEL PAIN

Heel pain represents a significant and hitherto intractable problem in podiatric and orthopaedic practice. The causes can be many and varied. As always, the cause must be established and, if systemic, suitably treated. However, much of the heel pain associated with calcaneal spur formation at the insertion of the plantar fascia, plantar fascitis, drag periostitis, and the loss of fibro-fatty tissue around the heel in the elderly, is not treated well or effectively. This leaves the patient in pain and the practitioner with a therapeutic puzzle.

I have found that with a very minor modification of the techniques of EVA orthosis manufacture, much relief can be given. The additional technique removes weight from the plantar surface of the calcaneus, and transfers it to the perimeter of the heel. The under surface of the heel is, if you like, allowed to float in the shoe. Using this technique along with the biomechanical control offered by the orthosis, ensures that heel pain due to the instances mentioned can at best be removed, and at worst significantly relieved.

Technique

1. The EVA orthosis is manufactured and finished as already described in Techniques I, II or III. However, the taper machined onto the outside edges of the heel, to allow a snug fit into the heel of the shoe, is adapted slightly. At this stage, slightly less of a taper is machined than would be expected (Fig. 9.1).

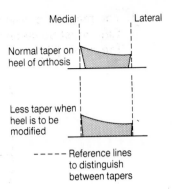

Medial　　　　Lateral

Normal taper on
heel of orthosis

Less taper when
heel is to be
modified

– – – – Reference lines
to distinguish
between tapers

Fig. 9.1

2. The orthosis is turned upside down and a line is drawn across its inferior surface, which corresponds to the same position as the anterior border of a normal heel post (Fig. 9.2).

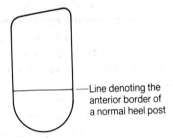

Line denoting the
anterior border of
a normal heel post

Fig. 9.2

3. Two marks are made on this line; one on either side. The positioning is critical and represents one-quarter of the width of the heel seat of the orthosis. The measurement is taken across the superior edges. Therefore, if the heel seat is 6 cm wide the marks will be made on the line, 1.5 cm in from the edge. (Fig. 9.3).

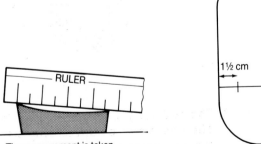

RULER

The measurement is taken
across the superior edges
of the heel seat of the
orthosis (measurement to the
outside edge of each side)

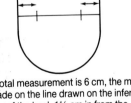

1½ cm　　1½ cm

If the total measurement is 6 cm, the marks
are made on the line drawn on the inferior
surface of the heel, 1½ cm in from the
sides

Fig. 9.3

4. The marks are now joined by drawing a 'U' shape around the heel. Care must be taken to maintain the correct width all the way around the heel. (Fig. 9.4).

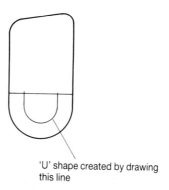

'U' shape created by drawing
this line

Fig. 9.4

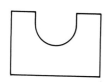

Fig. 9.5

5. A piece of EVA of 360 kg/m^3 density and large enough to cover the heel seat is chosen. It is economic to reduce the thickness to 6 mm. This is most easily achieved using a band-saw. It is then marked out in the 'U' shape required and the centre portion of the 'U' is removed on the band-saw. (A razor-sharp knife or scissors could be used.)
   This process leaves the shape shown in Figure 9.5.
6. Contact adhesive is now applied to the surfaces that require joining. Care must be taken to apply the glue only to the area on the orthosis that is to receive the extra material (Fig. 9.6).

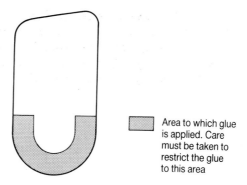

Area to which glue
is applied. Care
must be taken to
restrict the glue
to this area

Fig. 9.6

7. The additional EVA 'U' does not require heating prior to joining. The under surface of the orthosis, having already been ground to the correct posting angulation, will be entirely flat; the two flat surfaces will easily adhere.
8. Once attached, the additional material is ground to reduce it to approximately 3 mm in thickness (the actual thickness will increase in proportion to the weight of the patient but will not exceed 5

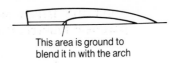

This area is ground to
blend it in with the arch

Fig. 9.7

mm.) Care must be taken not to alter the frontal plane posting angulation.

9. All that is then necessary is to continue the 'grinding out' of the
   arch area that was performed earlier to allow the orthosis to bend
   in the shoe; this should encompass the anterior edges of this additional material (Fig. 9.7).
10. The orthosis is now ready for issue.

INCREASED CONTROL AT THE SUB-TALAR JOINT

Firm control of the sub-talar joint function was hard to achieve when
initial experimentation began using EVA for the manufacture of accommodative orthoses. This is now overcome.

Technique

1. The orthosis is manufactured by any one of the methods already
   described, except that the sides are left at approximately 8 mm in
   thickness instead of being reduced to 3 mm in thickness.
2. The anterior border of the heel post is marked in pencil on the inferior surface of the orthosis (Fig. 9.8).

Anterior border of
heel post

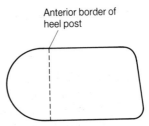

Fig. 9.8

3. A further line is drawn on the medial side of the orthosis to correspond to the tuberosity of the navicular (Fig. 9.9).

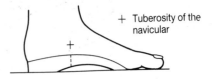

+ Tuberosity of the
navicular

Fig. 9.9

On the lateral side a line is drawn to correspond to the peroneal tubercle (Fig. 9.10).

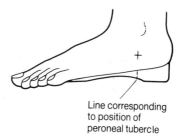

Line corresponding
to position of
peroneal tubercle

Fig. 9.10

4. The two lines marking the navicular and peroneal tubercle on the sides of the orthosis are joined by recessing the sides of the heel seat of the orthosis to 3 mm in thickness (Fig. 9.11).

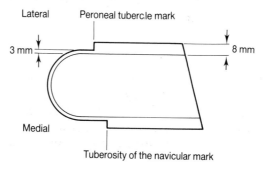

Fig. 9.11 View of orthosis from above.

5. The inferior surface of the heel is now also recessed but in the area of the post only; the anterior border line indicates the most distal part of this recess. It is recessed in from the sides to one-quarter of the width of the heel seat. The recess is 3 mm deep. The marking out procedure is the same as for step 3 of the heel floating technique just described (Fig. 9.12).

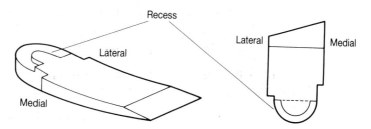

Fig. 9.12 View of inferior surface of orthosis.

The purpose of the recess is to allow for the moulding and insertion of a more rigid, controlling thermoplastic.

6. A strip of Subortholen or polypropylene of 3 mm thickness is cut to size. It must be wide enough to encompass the sides of the heel and then to fold underneath the heel seat and fit snugly into the recess which has been prepared for it. It is prepared by noting the point at which it will be required to bend from the sides of the heel to underneath the heel seat. To establish this a mark is made at either end of the material (Fig. 9.13).

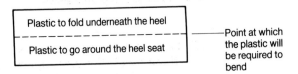

Fig. 9.13

The part of the plastic corresponding to the centre of the back of the heel is marked and then a similar marking is made on either side of the central mark at a point halfway around the curve both medially and laterally around the heel (Fig. 9.14).

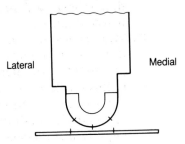

Fig. 9.14 View of inferior surface of orthosis.

When these marks have been made on the plastic, the bandsaw is used to remove two 'v' shapes from the area of plastic that is bent onto the inferior surface of the heel seat. A further two cuts are made in the plastic strip at the points corresponding to the changes in the lie of the recess (Fig. 9.15 A and B). This is to enable the plastic to be folded neatly into the recess without puckering.

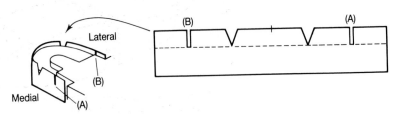

Fig. 9.15

Removing these two 'v' shaped 'cut outs' will prevent the pucker-ing that would otherwise inevitably occur when the plastic is bent around the heel and then down onto the inferior surface of the heel seat. Having cut out the 'v' shapes, a taper is put on either end of the plastic strip (Fig. 9.16).

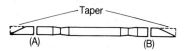

Fig. 9.16 Plastic strip from above.

7. Once cut to the correct size, the thermoplastic material is pos-itioned with the side tapers facing uppermost. It is sanded on this side and glue is applied, which is allowed to become 'touch' dry. The material is then placed in the oven to soften it. (A small electric grill is useful for heating such small pieces of plastic.)
8. While the material is being heated, glue is applied to the recess prepared on the orthosis. The orthosis is secured to the cast with masking tape and put to one side to allow the glue to dry.
9. By the time the thermoplastic has become mouldable, the glue on the orthosis will be dry. You must now put on a pair of heat-resistant gloves.
10. With gloves on, the thermoplastic is checked for mouldability and, if ready, is removed from the oven and inserted around the perimeter of the heel into the recess already made. Once secure in this position, one hand is used to apply pressure to it while the other hand is used to press the remainder of the material into the recess underneath the heel seat. Care must be taken when press-ing this area by hand not to cause unevenness. This will cause dis-comfort to the wearer. A small sheet of glass is useful for pressing the material firmly into the recess made for it. This ensures that the material is flat all around the inferior surface of the heel seat (Fig. 9.17).

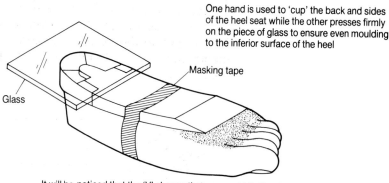

One hand is used to 'cup' the back and sides of the heel seat while the other presses firmly on the piece of glass to ensure even moulding to the inferior surface of the heel

Masking tape

Glass

It will be noticed that the 'V' shapes that were cut into the plastic close on moulding to join evenly

Fig. 9.17

11. Now the thermoplastic must be allowed to cool. Following this, the EVA along the sides of the orthosis which was left at approximately 8 mm wide is ground to the same level as the thermoplastic heel support (Fig. 9.18).

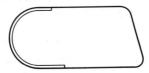

The sides of the orthosis are ground until they become flush with the reinforcing around the heel

Fig. 9.18 View of orthosis from above.

12. The orthosis may now be smoothed on the polisher to create an 'inside' bevel on the superior edge of the walls of the orthosis. This sympathetically blends the EVA into the firmer heel support (Fig. 9.19).

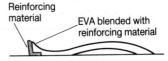

Reinforcing material

EVA blended with reinforcing material

Fig. 9.19 Sagittal cross-section of orthosis.

13. A covering material of choice may now be added.

Note

By encasing the EVA in the area of the heel, this modification helps to resist compression and remodelling of the material and thus produces a firmer, more durable platform for the heel.

If optimum control of the sub-talar joint is required of the orthosis, it is necessary to increase the height of the *reinforcing cup* around the heel. If this is the case, it is brought on the lateral side, just proximal to the base of the fifth metatarsal to a height just inferior to the peroneal tubercle. This height is extended right around the heel medially, to a point just proximal to the medial cuneiform. From these points distally, the sides of the orthosis are returned to the dimensions given in the section on 'marking out'. Care should be exercised when blending the EVA with the reinforcing heel cup so that the width of the orthosis is not increased (Fig. 19.20).

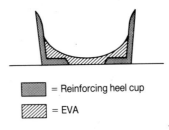

= Reinforcing heel cup

= EVA

Fig. 9.20

To achieve any greater control of the joint than this, the bracing must extend proximal to it in the form of a calliper or ankle-foot orthosis (AFO).

CONTROL OF SUB-TALAR JOINT FUNCTION WITH ADDITIONAL CUSHIONING

(This technique is of particular value when treating the arthritic patient.)

The technique has been partially dealt with already and centres around the blending of materials of differing therapeutic qualities prior to moulding. Most commonly, I blend three materials together. Starting from the inside of the orthosis outwards, these are (Fig. 9.21):

- 3 mm medium density Plastazote
- 3 mm closed-cell rubber or polyethylene foam
- 6 mm 260 or 360 EVA, depending on the weight of the patient.

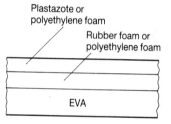

Plastazote or polyethylene foam

Rubber foam or polyethylene foam

EVA

Fig. 9.21

All three materials are stuck together prior to heating. I usually keep a number of these 'sandwiches' pre-stuck and cut to size in readiness. This saves manufacturing time. The material sandwich is heated in the oven until the EVA becomes mouldable.

The Plastazote side is then placed on the positive cast and the materials are pressed in the usual manner.

Once cooled, the EVA will maintain the correct shape, not only of itself but also of the other two materials.

It is ground by following any one of the three main manufacturing techniques, but can be modified in any way desired. It is a quick, relatively easy and very effective means of soft-based orthosis construction which has the added advantage of functional balancing and control.

10
Intrinsic posting

All the posting and methods of post application dealt with so far have related to attaching materials to the outside of the shell of the orthosis. These materials are then ground to the correct angle so that abnormal compensatory movement of the foot and limb at mid-stance is prevented. These posts, by way of definition, may be termed 'extrinsic' as they are attached to the outside, or exterior, of the shell of the orthosis.

However, it is possible to avoid the need for materials to be attached to the exterior of the shell. This is done by moulding the shell of the orthosis at its anterior border and the plantar surface of the heel, so that it becomes parallel with the ground while holding the foot at the correct frontal plane angulation.

Let us deal first with the intrinsic posting of the fore-foot, which is a concept many students find difficult to grasp. It becomes easier to assimiliate if you remove the thought of feet, and think for a moment of some methods of supporting a flat sheet of cardboard at a slightly inclined angle to a supporting surface. If you wish to raise the cardboard and support it at an angle, there are two ways in which this can be done.

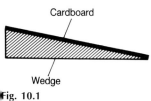

Cardboard

Wedge

Fig. 10.1

1. The first way is to put a wedge of material underneath the cardboard (Fig. 10.1).
2. The second way is to mark a point on one edge of the cardboard, which is set back the distance by which you wish to raise the material from the supporting surface. A diagonal line is then drawn across the material to meet the opposite corner (Fig. 10.2).

If the material is bent along the diagonal line and the edge distal to the bend is placed on the supporting surface, the sheet will, overall, be held at an angle. Try doing this with a piece of stiff cardboard.

These examples are conceptual, for the resemblance of the plantar surface of the foot to a flat piece of cardboard is not great. However, it is possible to relate the first method just described to the concept of extrinsic posting and the second method to that of intrinsic posting of the fore-foot.

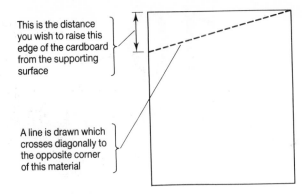

This is the distance you wish to raise this edge of the cardboard from the supporting surface

A line is drawn which crosses diagonally to the opposite corner of this material

Fig. 10.2

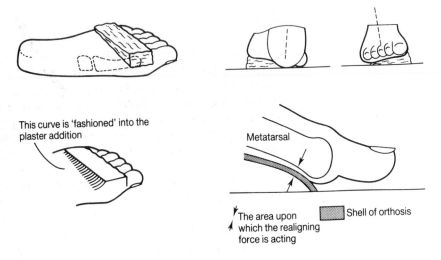

This curve is 'fashioned' into the plaster addition

Metatarsal

The area upon which the realigning force is acting

Shell of orthosis

Fig. 10.3

In reality, the alteration that must be made to the fore-foot of the positive cast involves the addition of sufficient plaster of Paris on the plantar surface of the metatarsophalangeal joints to hold the *cast* in the posting angle required (Fig. 10.3). When performed in the method to be described shortly, the effect on the shell when pressed is to put an exaggerated bend just proximal to the metatarsal heads. The increased convex curvature of the anterior border of the shell that is produced has the effect of realigning the skeletal structure of the foot in stance, and in so doing avoids the need for compensation.

With this method of 'posting', the alteration in the angle to the ground that it is necessary to achieve at the fore-foot, to prevent compensation, is built into the positive cast. This changes the shape of the distal one-third of the shell, which is curved to 'prop' up the required area of the foot. This overcomes the need to add additional material after pressing; the anterior border of the shell itself acts as the support, or post.

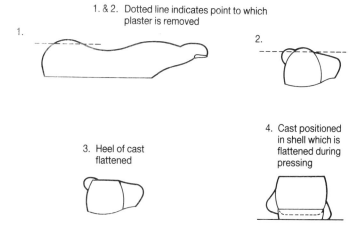

1. & 2. Dotted line indicates point to which plaster is removed

1.

2.

3. Heel of cast flattened

4. Cast positioned in shell which is flattened during pressing

Fig. 10.4

At the rear-foot the concept is slightly different and relates to the flattening out of a convex, and as such, a relatively unstable surface. Once more, for a moment, forget the foot and its dynamics and focus purely on concepts. Imagine that you have a wooden ball. Inherently this is unstable and will assume any position when allowed to move freely. However, if you hold the ball firmly and rub it on a sheet of sandpaper so as to flatten a significant proportion of one side of it, the ball will, if placed on the flattened side, develop stability.

The intrinsic posting of the rear-foot adopts this concept and requires therefore not the addition of plaster of Paris but removal, this being from the convex plantar surface of the heel. This can be done to develop stability at the required frontal plane angle (Fig. 10.4). Intrinsic posting of the fore-foot and rear-foot can be used independently or in conjunction with one another, depending on the therapeutic advantage that is sought.

POINTS TO CONSIDER WHEN DECIDING WHETHER TO USE INTRINSIC POSTS

FORE-FOOT

1. The angle of fore-foot anomaly which requires posting (i.e. the sum total of the frontal plane angulations minus any pronation allowance) cannot exceed 4 degrees, if this method of fore-foot posting is to be used. This is because the resulting angle of curvature of the anterior one-third of the shell of the orthosis would be excessive and would cause irritation and discomfort to the neck of the metatarsals that bear upon it (Fig. 10.5).
   Therefore, in practice, the maximum valgus anomaly of the fore-foot that can be intrinsically posted is 4 degrees. However, the maximum varus anomaly, when computed by the method described in Chap-

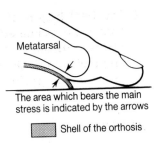

Metatarsal

The area which bears the main
stress is indicated by the arrows

Shell of the orthosis

Fig. 10.5

ter 1, will be 8 degrees because 4 degrees are removed from fore-
foot posting computation to allow for sub-talar pronation (assuming
sufficient range of motion is available at the sub-talar joint). This
means that the *actual* maximum angular change built into the fore-
foot of the shell will be only 4 degrees.

2. If the fore-foot posting angle required is greater than 2 degrees, intrinsic posting of the fore-foot can only be considered if rigid shell
materials are to be used. Materials of a flexible or semi-flexible nature will bend under body weight when the ground reactionary
forces are exerted upon them during stance. If they bend and flatten during stance, then the controlling effect of the orthosis will be
nullified.

3. When used on heavy people or people who pursue strenuous activities (i.e. long-distance running), the anterior border of the shell
of the orthosis can cause a depression in the inner-sole of the shoe,
owing to the acute angle at which they abut. This reduces the effectiveness of the biomechanical control. It is far more marked, of
course, if the inner-sole of the shoe is at all soft.

4. The accuracy of your work is critical when employing this method
of fore-foot posting because you are actually altering the shape of
the positive cast. Once the plaster addition has been made, no alteration in the length of the shell of the orthosis is possible; nor can
the angle of the fore-foot post be changed. (Reducing the angle of
the fore-foot post on the shell will, of course, also shorten the length
of the shell, and vice versa.)

REAR-FOOT

1. Because this method of posting slightly flattens the plantar surface
of the heel of the shell, consideration should be given to this inherent feature. When treatment is being administered to relieve the
adaptive stresses which accumulate to produce pain associated with
a calcaneal spur or drag periostitis, a therapeutic advantage can
sometimes be gained by maintaining the convexity of the plantar
contours of the heel.
In this instance, intrinsic posting of the rear-foot should be avoided.

2. The heel height of the shoe in which the orthosis is to be worn should be examined carefully to ensure that the sagittal angulation of the intrinsic post is correct. This is particularly important when employing intrinsic rear-foot posting since irreparable change will be made to the positive cast.

GENERAL

Intrinsic posting, if performed carefully, is effective. It also does have the advantage of there being no material stuck to the shell which is at risk of avulsing during use. However, this advantage does not necessarily outweigh some of the inherent problems associated with this method of posting. As always, skill and thereapeutic acumen must be exercised if intrinsic posting is to be used successfully. It is advantageous to develop some practice and expertise in extrinsic posting techniques and therapeutic possibilities before this slightly more technical exercise is attempted.

INTRINSIC POSTING TECHNIQUE

Tools/materials required

Rubber bowl
Three 'panel-pin' nails (per foot)
Plaster of Paris powder
Spatula
Hammer
Sand-Screen abrasive cloth
Grease-proof paper
Tractograph
Material for heel raise (cork sheeting is ideal).

FORE-FOOT POSTING

Method

1. The negative foot cast is produced by neutral casting, in exactly the same manner as has already been described. The positive cast once poured is allowed to set and is then removed from the negative cast and the rear-foot bisection line is checked and reinforced if necessary.
2. The bisections of the first and fifth metarsophalangeal joints are marked by either of the methods described on pages 40–41. At this point, the technique varies according to the frontal plane deformity being dealt with.

Varus deformity at the fore-foot

If dealing with a varus deformity of the fore-foot, be it 'pure' or 'compounded' (i.e. a true inversion discrepancy between the fore- and rear-foot or an inversion of the fore-foot created by an accumulation of the frontal plane deformities of the whole limb), the following instructions must be adhered to:

3. A nail is driven into the positive cast at a point 0.5 cm proximal to the fifth metatarsophalangeal joint. It is driven in at a point midway between the joint and the lateral border of the foot (Fig. 10.6). It is inserted until it is level with the highest point on this side of the foot. This can be *examined* by positioning the cast the right way up on the bench with the heel raised to the required height and angled at the correct frontal plane angulation. A check is then made to see if the most prominent area of the plantar surface of the fifth metatarsal head is flush with the bench top (Fig. 10.7).

4. A point 1 cm proximal to the bisection of the first metatarsophalangeal joint is now marked and a nail driven in at this point. One very important detail must be stressed. If you have worked through this text you will have become familiar with grinding extrinsic posts, the rear-foot first followed by the fore-foot, which is *reduced by the necessary amount to allow pronation at the sub-talar joint*. This reduction in the fore-foot posting angle must not be overlooked when intrinsically posting the cast for an inversion deformity.

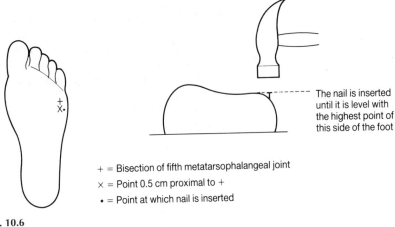

The nail is inserted until it is level with the highest point of this side of the foot

+ = Bisection of fifth metatarsophalangeal joint
x = Point 0.5 cm proximal to +
• = Point at which nail is inserted

Fig. 10.6

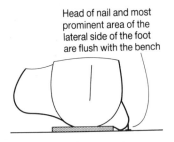

Head of nail and most prominent area of the lateral side of the foot are flush with the bench

Fig. 10.7

However, because the fore-foot is being posted *before* the rear-foot in this posting method, it is easy to forget this important detail.

Therefore, the pronation allowance is deducted from the rear-foot angle, as explained on pages 84 and 92. This will reduce the angulation of the fore-foot angle by a corresponding amount. The nail being driven into this side of the cast is inserted until the cast is angled correctly when positioned on the bench (Fig. 10.8).

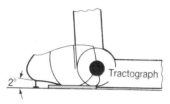

In this example the fore-foot is *actually* posted in only 2° of inversion. To set this accurately the rear-foot bisection line is used and is everted by 4° from 90°. This will reduce the fore-foot measurement by a corresponding amount.

Fig. 10.8 Material to be used: 3 mm Rohadur—6° fore-foot varus—rear-foot 90°.

The correct positioning of the cast is checked by placing a tractograph against the rear-foot bisection line, after having deducted the required pronation allowance at the fore-foot from the overall frontal plane rear-foot angle.

Valgus deformity at fore-foot

5. When preparing the cast for intrinsic posting of the fore-foot in this frontal plane deformity, the first nail is inserted on the medial side of the cast at a point 1 cm proximal to the bisection of the first metatarsophalangeal joint. It is driven in sufficiently far so that, when the cast is positioned on the bench at the required frontal plane angulation and the heel is raised to the required height, the first metatarsophalangeal joint is flush with the supporting surface (Fig. 10.9).

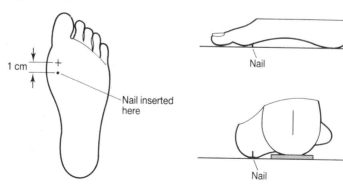

Note that the head of the nail and the first metatarsophalangeal joint are both flush with the supporting surface

Fig. 10.9

6. The second nail is driven into the cast at the point 0.5 cm proximal to the fifth metatarsophalangeal joint. It is driven in until the rear-foot bisection line corresponds to the frontal plane measurement required.

Remember that in valgus deformities of the fore-foot the posting of the fore-foot is absolute. Remember *why* you are supporting this fore-foot anomaly. In general terms it is to maintain the mid-tarsal joint in a locked position. From now on, the technique of intrinsically posting the fore-foot is similar regardless of the frontal plane deformity being treated clinically.

7. A bowl of plaster is mixed and allowed to set until it has the consistency of soft ice-cream. The mixing of this plaster can be done before marking-out and inserting the nails in the fore-foot, so that some time is allowed for setting. (Polyfilla or any suitable household filler is ideal for the purpose of intrinsically posting the fore-foot.) Remember to soak the positive cast well before adding any additional plaster.

8. Plaster of this thick consistency is added to the cast in the area overlying the metatarsophalangeal joints, occupying a space just proximal to the metal nails and distal to the joints themselves. The addition should span the whole width of the fore-foot in this area and be about 2 mm proud of the nail heads (Fig. 10.10).

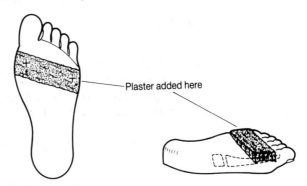

Plaster added here

Fig. 10.10

9. A piece of grease-proof paper 12 cm × 6 cm is placed on a flat bench or board. The size is not critical, but it should have at least the same surface area as the prospective 'post'. The positive cast is then turned the right way up and positioned so that the plaster addition is on the grease-proof paper and the heel is raised to the required height (Fig. 10.11).

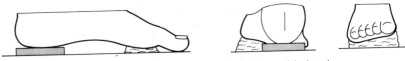

Greaseproof paper placed between the added plaster and the bench

Fig. 10.11

10. The fore-foot is firmly pressed down to squeeze away any excess plaster, until the heads of the two nails come into contact with the supporting surface. It is better to press down firmly rather than to slide the cast from side to side. The sliding motion sometimes fractures the partially set, plaster of Paris addition. Once positioned correctly, the cast is left to allow the plaster to set.

11. Once the added plaster has set, the cast can be handled and is turned upside down. The grease-proof paper is peeled away to reveal the heads of the two nails which should now be visible. These are joined by drawing a line between them (Fig. 10.12).

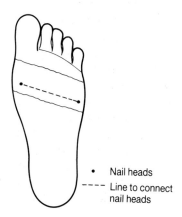

•   Nail heads
---- Line to connect
     nail heads

Fig. 10.12

12. A hack-saw placed beside this line and immediately proximal to it is used to saw down through the added plaster to the level of the original cast. The saw is held perpendicular to the inferior surface of the added plaster (Fig. 10.13).

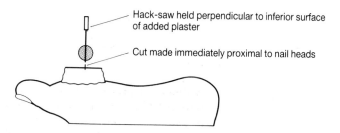

Hack-saw held perpendicular to inferior surface of added plaster

Cut made immediately proximal to nail heads

Fig. 10.13

13. The added plaster which is proximal to the saw cut is removed (Fig. 10.14).

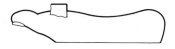

Fig. 10.14

14. The positive cast is now modified to allow for the tissue adaptation of weight bearing. The modification in nearly all aspects is identical to that already described in Chapter 5. The only difference in the technique here is that the plaster used to modify the medial and lateral arches of the cast must be fashioned sympathetically to form a gradual curve, reaching from two-thirds of the way down the metatarsals to meet the inferior surface of the fore-foot post (Fig. 10.15).

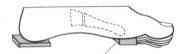

The modification plaster is fashioned sympathetically to form a gradual curve which meets the inferior surface of the intrinsic fore-foot post

Fig. 10.15

This curving prevents any abrupt changes in the sagittal angulation of the fore-foot from causing irritation to the plantar surface of the fore-foot of the wearer. It inevitably means that some plaster must be added to the cast the whole way across the fore-foot in order that a suitable curve is created (Fig. 10.16).

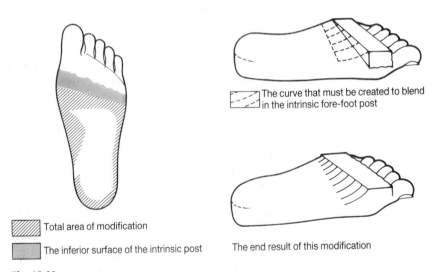

The curve that must be created to blend in the intrinsic fore-foot post

Total area of modification

The inferior surface of the intrinsic post

The end result of this modification

Fig. 10.16

At this point, if the rear-foot is to be posted extrinsically a final smoothing of the cast is carried out and it is allowed to dry; it is then marked out in the normal manner and the shell is pressed.

When grinding the shell to the required shape, the anterior border which is clearly visible is ground on its inferior surface to lie flush,

Sagittal section through the shell of an
orthosis

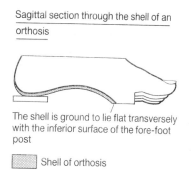

The shell is ground to lie flat transversely
with the inferior surface of the fore-foot
post

▨ Shell of orthosis

Fig. 10.17

transversely with the platform or post created by the plaster that was added (Fig. 10.17).

The shell, having been fashioned and polished in the normal way, is then ready to have the rear-foot post attached. This is performed as described in Chapter 7. Remember when doing this, if a varus anomaly of the fore-foot has been posted, to return the rear-foot to its correct frontal plane angulation which was reduced by the necessary pronatory allowance when the fore-foot post was created.

INTRINSIC REAR-FOOT POSTING

As explained in the introduction to this chapter, there is an alternative to the 'extrinsic' post as a means of gaining control at the rear-foot. To do this, a further modification is made to the positive cast; this is loosely covered in the introduction to this chapter, and involves the removal of some of the plaster of Paris from the plantar surface of the heel of the positive foot cast.

This method of posting is useful for controlling simple anomalies in frontal plane angulations of a limb. (The control gained at the rear-foot acts along similar lines to a heel meniscus, a well tried and successful therapy, but one which is difficult to accomplish well.) It does, however, remove some of the many therapeutic possibilities available to the clinician when considering the rear-foot posting of an orthosis, in particular the blending of shock absorption with control of the sub-talar joint. Sub-talar control from an intrinsic rear-foot post is gained using the material of the shell only, and as such, the density of the shell material governs the therapeutic qualities of the rear-foot post of the orthosis. Consideration must be given to the needs of the wearer.

This method of gaining control of the rear-foot is *not* the one of choice in the following situations:

1. When it is therapeutically advantageous to maintain the convex dome of the plantar surface of heel when treating the symptoms of a calcaneal spur.

2. When, in treating the foot affected by rheumatoid arthritis, control of the sub-talar joint and shock absorption at heel strike are the therapeutic requirements.
3. When manufacturing accommodative EVA orthoses.
4. When lesions on the heel require specific redistribution within the orthosis.

However, this method *is* particularly useful when:

- The heel-counter of the shoe lacks depth, as is common in some women's shoes (and nowadays in some fashion shoes for men). Because no extra material is added to the heel of the orthosis and some of the convex dome of the heel is reduced, the risk of lifting the heel out of the shoe is minimised.
- The therapeutic requirement of the orthosis is limited to controlling simple frontal plane anomalies.

Note

This method can be used in conjunction with extrinsic rear-foot posting on a 50/50 basis—aproximately 30% of the plantar curve of the heel being removed but the main control is gained from the extrinsic post. This has the advantage of reducing the depth of the heel-seat of the orthosis and, in so doing, reducing the likelihood of the heel of the wearer being lifted out of the shoe. Used in this way, some of the disadvantages outlined can be overcome. Therapies are as much an art as a science and, as such, a 'feel' will be developed in using the intrinsic/extrinsic rear-foot post blend to the best advantage of your patient.

Materials/equipment required

These are the same as are required for intrinsically posting the fore-foot.

Method

This method of gaining control of the rear-foot can be used regardless of whether the fore-foot is to have an extrinsic post added or has already had an intrinsic post built into the cast. Therefore, it can be used independently to either of the fore-foot posting methods. If it is to be used in conjunction with an intrinsic post at the fore-foot, the fore-foot post is applied first and the cast modified before the rear-foot posting technique is executed. If an extrinsic fore-foot post is to be applied to the shell of the orthosis, the positive cast is modified and the intrinsic rear-foot post ground into it. The shell is then pressed. The extrinsic fore-foot post is then applied to the shell in the normal manner.

Technique

1. A nail is driven into the plantar surface of either the first or fifth

metatarsophalangeal joint of the cast, depending on whether a varus or valgus anomaly of the fore-foot or rear-foot exists.

(If a valgus anomaly of the fore-foot has already been posted intrinsically there is no need to insert a nail under the fifth metatarsophalangeal joint.)

The nail is driven into the cast until when, by placing the positive cast on a flat surface, the rear-foot bisection line is held at the cor-

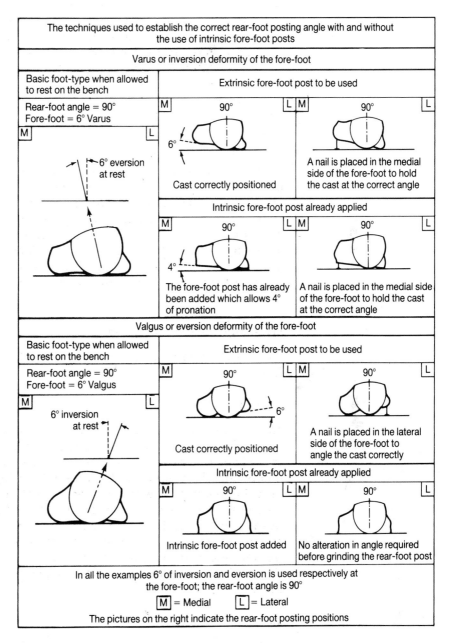

Fig. 10.18

rect angulation. Remember this will mean that, if you have already intrinsically posted a varus anomaly of the fore-foot, the rear-foot bisection line will be returned to a position which is inverted 4 degrees more than the fore-foot because of the allowance made at the fore-foot *of an orthosis* for pronation at the sub-talar joint. This of course, will only relate to inversion deformities of the fore-foot *and* when sufficient range of motion is available to allow pronation to occur (Fig. 10.18).

2. Once the rear-foot angle has been established correctly, the heel of the orthosis is raised the required amount to allow for the heel height of the shoe. On the piece of material used for this raise is placed some Sand-Screen abrasive cloth. (Cork sheeting is ideal for raising the heels of these casts, as it prevents the abrasive cloth from slipping during the next phase of the work.)

3. The positive cast is held with the fore-foot positioned securely on the supporting surface. It is supported at the correct angle by the nail already inserted. It is then rubbed forwards and backwards in order to remove some plaster of Paris from the plantar surface of the heel of the positive cast.

This process is continued until approximately three-quarters of the surface area of the plantar surface of the heel is removed. (Fig. 10.19).

Note: In more significant frontal plane deformities of the rear-foot, care should be taken not to remove plaster beyond the area of the plantar surface of the heel. The removal of plaster must be stopped once the inferior surface of the curve representing the border be-

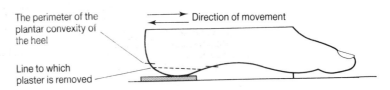

The perimeter of the plantar convexity of the heel

Line to which plaster is removed

Direction of movement

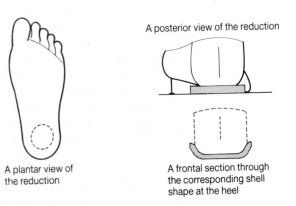

A plantar view of the reduction

A posterior view of the reduction

A frontal section through the corresponding shell shape at the heel

Fig. 10.19

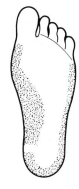

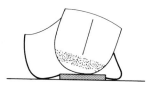

This will mean that it is not possible to use intrinsic posting at the rear-foot in severe frontal plane deformities due to an insufficiently large surface area of the post resulting from the grinding procedure

 Area of additional plaster applied as a modification to the positive cast

Removal of plaster from the plantar surface of the heel must be stopped once the inferior margin of the modification plaster is reached

Fig. 10.20

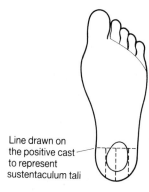

Line drawn on the positive cast to represent sustentaculum tali

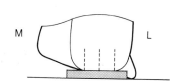

M L

Fig. 10.21

tween the plantar surface of the heel and either the medial or lateral sides of the foot is reached. This will normally be indicated by reaching the most plantar limit of the modification plaster added to the perimeter of the heel (Fig. 10.20).

4. If dealing with varus anomalies, it is now necessary to remove a little plaster from the medial side of the plantar surface of the heel to allow the orthosis to rock in pronation.

It is easier to accomplish this correctly if the plantar surface of the heel is divided transversely into quarters (Fig. 10.21).

Plaster is removed from the most medial quarter only as far distally as the reference line drawn down from sustentaculum tali. The convexity of this quarter should be flattened to enable the fulcrum created by the edge of its most plantar margin and the medial edge of the rear-foot post to function effectively and to allow the orthosis to tip medially in pronation (Fig. 10.22).

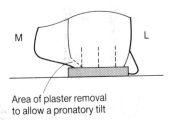

M   L

Area of plaster removal
to allow a pronatory tilt

Fig. 10.22

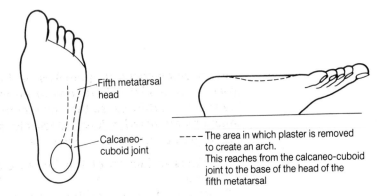

-Fifth metatarsal
 head

-Calcaneo-
 cuboid joint

---- The area in which plaster is removed
to create an arch.
This reaches from the calcaneo-cuboid
joint to the base of the head of the
fifth metatarsal

Fig. 10.23

This flattening must be sympathetically blended in with the cast superiorly, distally and proximally.

5. The last procedure to be accomplished, is the removal of a little plaster along the plantar surface of the fifth ray so that a pronatory force (locking force) is maintained at the mid-tarsal joint. This creates a slight arching of this border, and is particularly important when only a small convex curvature of the heel is present. When this is the case, the flattening of the plantar surface of the heel to create the 'post' removes the proximal end of the lateral longitudinal arch. This must be restored in order to maintain the pronatory force on the mid-tarsal joint (Fig. 10.23).

Once the cast has had a final smoothing, it is allowed to dry. The shell may then be pressed. The rear-foot post will be incorporated in it and, if this is all that is required by way of posting, the shell may be ground and polished and dispensed.

If an extrinsic fore-foot post is required, this may now be stuck on and machined. If required, an intrinsic fore-foot post will of course have been added to the cast before the modification and intrinsic rear-foot post was added.

11

Unusual shapes for shells of orthoses

Certain biomechanical anomalies of the lower limb and certain foot-types require slight alterations to be made to the standard shape of the shells of orthoses, so that the therapeutic objectives are met. These situations are listed below collectively, and will be explained individually in greater detail later. They are:

1. When abduction of the fore-foot occurs distal to the mid-tarsal joint
2. When adduction of the fore-foot occurs distal to the mid-tarsal joint
3. When increased control of the calcaneus is required. This can be when a restricted *painful* range of motion is present at the sub-talar joint, in conditions of hypermobility or when large alterations are necessary in the frontal plane angulation of the calcaneus. (In order to control these situations most effectively, shoe modifications and/or callipers are often required in addition to the orthosis)
4. When a rigid plantar-flexed first ray is present
5. In-toeing and out-toeing gait patterns

Let us now deal with these situations in detail.

ABDUCTION OF THE FOOT DISTAL TO THE MID-TARSAL JOINT

This situation can arise from a number of causes; the more common of these are:

a. Hypermobility, particularly in children, resulting in excessive pronation at the sub-talar joint. When this occurs, an abductory force is placed on the foot distal to the mid-tarsal joint, owing to the forward line of progression of the body during gait, and the medial movement of the talus as the leg rotates internally (Fig. 11.1).
   If this condition remains untreated, a long-term structural deformity results and a mid-tarsal fault becomes evident as an uncorrectable abduction of the fore-foot. The overall treatment of this

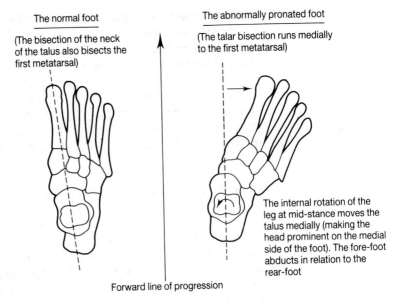

The normal foot

(The bisection of the neck of the talus also bisects the first metatarsal)

The abnormally pronated foot

(The talar bisection runs medially to the first metatarsal)

The internal rotation of the leg at mid-stance moves the talus medially (making the head prominent on the medial side of the foot). The fore-foot abducts in relation to the rear-foot

Forward line of progression

Fig. 11.1

anomaly is not in the brief of this text, but if orthoses are required as part of the therapy plan, alterations to the shape of the shell of the orthosis must be made; these will be explained shortly.

b. Compensatory changes in the foot owing to a restriction of internal rotation at the hip joint because of osteo-arthritis, or congenital muscular or skeletal deformities. Increased external torsion within the long bones of the leg may also cause this foot deformity.

c. Spasms of the peronei, a weak posterior tibial muscle or a tight Achilles tendon. These causes, individually or collectively, may impose forces on the fore-foot during gait. An equinus foot with a weak posterior tibial muscle and/or strong peronei, or any condition in which the body weight moves forward when this muscular imbalance is present, may result in the fore-foot abducting relative to the rear-foot.

d. Structural changes owing to arthrodesis of the sub-talar joint, either surgically produced or by the bony union known as talocalcaneal bar, or as a result of arthritis.

Regardless of the cause, if orthoses are to be used in the treatment plan, the information that follows is important.

If this condition is present in a child up to 7 years of age, when the cause is hypermobility or ligamentous laxity, the segmental interrelationship of the foot can be corrected when producing the negative cast. This method of casting has already been explained in Chapter 3. Because the architecture of the foot is restored during the negative casting procedure, no modification is required to the positive cast other than making good any imperfections to the surface.

When abduction of the fore-foot relative to the rear-foot has become a structural osseous anomaly, it is very difficult to alter the transverse plane relationship of the rear-foot and fore-foot by means of orthoses. This is because the reactive force produced by the orthosis on the tissues of the foot becomes too severe to bear. Therefore, no correction is made while taking the negative cast, which is performed in the way already described for the adult. The orthotic alteration is made to the shell alone, although the underlying medical condition and/or biomechanical anomaly must be diagnosed and treated.

ALTERATION TO THE SHELL OF THE ORTHOSIS

In all cases of abduction of the foot distal to the mid-tarsal joint, whether this has been corrected when casting or not, the shell of the orthosis must be extended laterally to reach around and up the lateral side of the foot. The high lateral flange that is produced maintains the correct alignment of the foot in a child and, in maintaining this corrected architecture, prevents long-term abnormal adaptations while sufficient muscle strength or phasic muscle balance is gained. In the adult or skeletally mature foot, such alteration prevents deterioration of the deformity and, importantly, the tendency the foot has to slide off the orthosis laterally during gait.

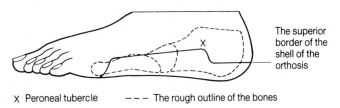

X Peroneal tubercle   – – – The rough outline of the bones

The superior border of the shell of the orthosis

Fig. 11.2 The shape of the lateral side of the orthosis when control of abduction of the fore-foot is required.

The alteration in shell shape is as follows. The medial side of the shell and heel cup are machined to the normal dimensions. They continue as such around to the lateral side of the foot until a point just proximal to the peroneal tubercle is reached. At this point, the height of the lateral side of the orthosis is raised until it is 3–5 mm inferior to the peroneal tubercle (the difference in distance from the peroneal tubercle will depend on the size of the foot). It is then extended at this height distally, until it is between 3 and 5 mm proximal to the head of the fifth metatarsal. At this point, the shell is machined in a cyma shape to descend to meet the lateral side of the anterior border of the shell of the orthosis, which corresponds to its normal dimension (Fig. 11.2). Remember, when making this orthosis for a child you must allow for the normal development of plantar-flexion of the first ray (p. 30).

Note

If this alteration is being performed in a case of restricted internal rotation at the hip joint owing to osteo-arthritis, the foot should also be examined to see the extent of the range of motion available at the sub-talar joint. The relaxed calcaneal stance measurement may indicate that the calcaneus is everted to the full extent of the eversion capabilities of this joint, especially if there is flexion of the knee and abduction of the whole foot. However, if the joint is mobile and has an adequate ability to invert, much relief can be gained from the symptoms of pain in the hip by holding the calcaneus in an inverted position on the orthosis. By inverting the calcaneus, the leg is externally rotated. If the range of motion of the foot is controlled, it is also possible to control the range of motion at the hip joint. This can be achieved by reducing the amount of pronation available at the sub-talar joint by posting the foot in an inverted position. In doing this, the degree of internal rotation that is required within the leg and hips, to stabilise the foot on the ground at mid-stance, is reduced. The range of motion of the hip is thus altered, enabling it to begin its cycle from a more externally rotated position. Therefore, the position at which internal rotation 'peaks' at mid-stance is also altered. The relief of stress at the hip joint that this achieves, does in my experience give significant relief from pain to people who suffer this disabling condition.

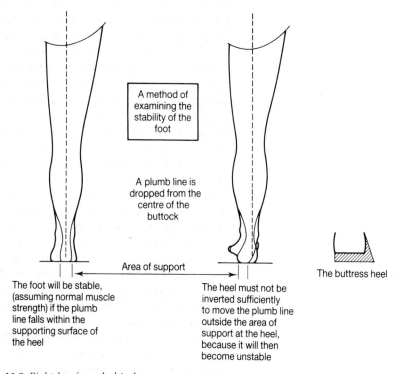

A method of examining the stability of the foot

A plumb line is dropped from the centre of the buttock

Area of support

The buttress heel

The foot will be stable, (assuming normal muscle strength) if the plumb line falls within the supporting surface of the heel

The heel must not be inverted sufficiently to move the plumb line outside the area of support at the heel, because it will then become unstable

Fig. 11.3 Right leg from behind.

You should remember three things when attempting this therapy:

- Do not invert the calcaneus to a position of instability, whereby the centre of gravity of the body falls outside (laterally) the area of support of the heel during mid-stance (Fig. 11.3). (Unless the heel counter of the shoe is stiffened and a buttress heel is applied to the shoe which moves the area of support laterally, and/or a boot is worn. A calliper can be used to provide the necessary support if desired.)
- Provide a 4 degree pronation allowance in the orthosis to prevent fracture of the material and allow motion at the sub-talar joint.
- Impress upon the patient that this treatment must stop if or when hip replacement surgery is performed. However, the results of such valuable surgery may be improved if the mechanics of the limb are examined thoroughly afterwards. Good results are sustainable both pre-operatively and post-operatively if a sound working relationship is enjoyed with the patient's orthopaedic surgeon.

ADDUCTION OF THE FOOT DISTAL TO THE MID-TARSAL JOINT

This situation can arise from a number of causes; the more common of these are:

a. *Talipes equinovarus*: this congenital condition, where the foot assumes a position of plantar-flexion, inversion and adduction, is invariably treated in the infant soon after birth. Many books have been written and many theories formed on all aspects of this condition, and I do not intend to go into these here. However, what is apparent is that having followed a full regime of treatment, which may often include orthopaedic surgery, the deformity that commonly remains is the inversion and adduction of the fore-foot distal to the mid-tarsal joint. This may be caused by, among many other things, a weakness of the peronei, these having been over-stretched by the initial deformity; or by the plantar-flexion of the first ray, which on heel-lift inverts the fore-foot dramatically just as it is subjected to the forces of propulsive thrust. This, combined with the forward direction of movement and the rotation occurring in the leg and hip, places an adductory force on the fore-foot, because of the opposite ground reaction. This is further aggravated by a strong tibialis posterior. It may be a combination of these things along with an over-pull of tibialis anterior during the swing phase of gait which helps to maintain the deformity. The podiatric orthotic treatment of this condition is fascinating, but in this section I intend only to describe a modification to the shape of the shell of an orthosis which helps to limit the adduction and inversion.

b. The shell modification I will explain shortly is also valuable in controlling the relative adduction of the fore-foot on the rear-foot in conditions such as pes cavus and metatarsus adductus. Furthermore, it is valuable in any condition that results in a gravitational drop-foot, such as multiple sclerosis, diabetis, polio (though this disease is selective, and which muscles are paralysed will depend totally on which anterior motor horns are affected), leprosy and Charcot-Marie-Tooth disease (where, commonly, an inverted, adducted fore-foot is seen, owing to the intrinsic muscle atrophy which later spreads to the peronei. This allows an over-pull of the tibialis posterior.). Also in cases of muscle atrophy, dorsiflexion of the toes on heel lift, particularly the first toe, produces a windlass effect on the plantar fascia which pulls on and plantar-flexes the first ray, causing further inversion of the fore-foot. A cerebrovascular accident and Parkinson's disease can cause adduction of the whole limb. The two conditions are of different aetiology: the stroke causes adduction by loss of muscle power, Parkinson's disease by rigidity of muscle tone.

The conditions listed as causing either abduction or adduction of the fore-foot are offered as a sample, in an effort to alert your mind to some of the more involved aspects of orthotic management, and to the importance of a thorough diagnosis and understanding of a patient's problem before orthoses are included in the treatment plan.

MODIFICATIONS REQUIRED

The modifications to the shape of the shell or casting procedures are as follows, and are divided into two categories:

(i)   The casting and shell modification required when the only element of deformity is an adduction of the fore-foot distal to the mid-tarsal Joint. This is also useful in treating mild pes cavus

(ii)   The casting modification required in the condition of metatarsus adductus.

Modifications required in the treatment of an adducted fore-foot

Examine the foot carefully and note, if present, the degree of plantar flexion of the first ray and/or the amount of frontal plane deformity of the fore-foot.

The child

Once again, when casting for the child under 7 years of age the adduction of the fore-foot can easily be reduced while producing the semi-weight-bearing negative cast. The correction is achieved while casting by holding the heel from behind with one hand, with the finger or thumb extending on the lateral side of the foot, no further than the distal edge of the calcaneus. The other hand is laid, palm downwards, over the dorsum of the foot with the thumb placed on the medial side of the first metatarsal head. With the heel held firmly and in the desired

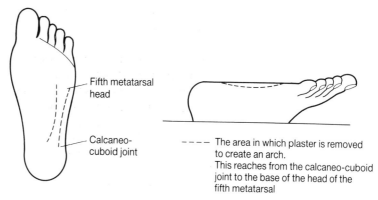

Fifth metatarsal head

Calcaneo-cuboid joint

- - - - The area in which plaster is removed to create an arch.
This reaches from the calcaneo-cuboid joint to the base of the head of the fifth metatarsal

Fig. 11.4

frontal plane angle, pressure is applied to the head of the first metatarsal in the direction of abduction, until the fore-foot is in the required position. This position is maintained until the plaster is set. When doing this, there is often a tendency for the metatarsals to bunch up in a convex curve dorsally as pressure is applied on the medial side of the fore-foot. If the hand has been placed over the dorsum of the foot, palm downwards, gentle pressure can be applied in a plantar direction to flatten and splay the metatarsals. When satisfied with the negative cast you have produced, the positive cast can be poured and allowed to set. One modification is required to be performed on the positive cast, and that is to remove plaster on the plantar surface of the cast to produce a concave curve along the line of the fifth metatarsal. This is similar to the modification performed on the plantar surface of the positive cast when intrinsic posting is used at the rear-foot. It is done so that a locking (pronatory) force is applied to the mid-tarsal joint when the child is standing on the orthosis. This is very important in order to improve the function of the foot and to help reduce the functional stresses which are one element in the production of the adduction (Fig. 11.4).

Having done this, the positive cast can be marked out as follows: The anterior border of the orthosis follows the normal dimensions of all juvenile functional orthoses, accounting for first ray motion as necessary. The lateral border follows the normal line proximally from the anterior border, until the fifth metatarsal/cuboid articulation is reached. At this point it curves up onto the lateral side of the foot until it is 3–5 mm inferior to the peroneal tubercle. This height is maintained around the heel and distally along the medial side of the foot to a point 3–5 mm proximal to the head of the first metatarsal. At this point it drops in a cyma shape to meet the medial side of the anterior border of the shell of the orthosis (Fig. 11.5).

The shell is then pressed and machined to the marked-out shape, and the rear-foot stabilising post applied.

Note: This orthosis is assisted in its action if a relatively straight-lasted shoe is worn (or boot, if significant control is required at the sub-talar

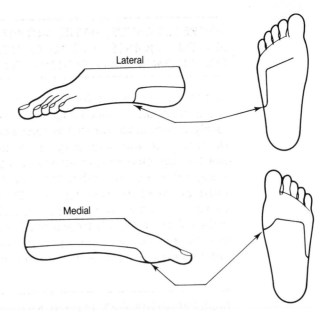

Fig. 11.5

joint). The shoe may require a 'buttress' heel (see p. 154) and the sole extended on the lateral side to move the moment arm of this additional and useful lever. The lateral extension of the sole and heel tends to increase the eversional force on the calcaneus and sub-talar joint.

The adult

If, in the adult, the adduction of the fore-foot is flexible because of muscle paralysis or atrophy, some correction can be achieved during the negative casting procedure. This is then best done in a semi-weight-bearing position, as for the child. In this case, the cast modification and shell adaptations are followed exactly as described for the child. If the adduction is due to a rigid deformity, no correction can be achieved on casting. This is then performed by the normal method explained for the adult. In the case we are considering, the modification of the positive cast is performed in the normal way but the dimensions of the shell of the orthosis follow those described for the child. This helps to prevent further deformity.

Modifications required in the condition of metatarsus adductus

The shape of the shell is exactly the same as the orthosis for the adducted fore-foot in a child. There is a minor difference in the casting procedure, whereby the fingers or thumb of the hand holding the calcaneus are moved distally on the lateral side to hold the cuboid as well. An abductory force is then applied to the medial side of the first metatarsal, as has already been described, and held until the cast is set.

SEVERE PES CAVUS, SEVERE ARTHRITIC DISEASE OF THE ANKLE AND SUB-TALAR JOINTS, AND ALL CONDITIONS WHICH HAVE RESULTED IN A GRAVITATIONAL FOOT DROP

In these situations, a foot orthosis which must be designed to meet the functional, biomechanical and therapeutic needs of the patient is rarely sufficient to control the forces causing pain or tending to produce deformity. In the case of gravitational foot drop, a foot orthosis cannot be expected to control the plantar flexion of the foot. A calliper designed to control either the frontal and/or sagittal plane deformity must be used in conjunction with the orthosis. There are many of these, the most cosmetically appealing of which is the 'ankle–foot orthosis' made of polypropylene. These orthoses are described in texts listed under Further Reading; the shoe modifications that are required are also described in texts listed in this section.

RIGID PLANTAR-FLEXED FIRST RAY

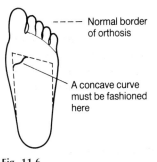

Normal border of orthosis

A concave curve must be fashioned here

Fig. 11.6

Positive cast modifications in the condition of plantar-flexed first ray have been described in Chapter 5. However, when the first ray is plantar-flexed and is rigid, the anterior border of the shell of the orthosis must be altered to accommodate the distal end of the first metatarsal. The medial side of the anterior border is machined in a concave curve to allow this area of the bone to sit comfortably. If this is not done, the pressure applied by the anterior border of the orthosis will be unbearable (Fig. 11.6).

Following the shell modification, the biomechanics may be treated in compliance with the clinical measurements.

IN-TOEING AND OUT-TOEING GAIT PATTERNS

To understand the concept behind the mode of action of orthoses used to treat the particular gait anomalies of in-toeing and out-toeing, we must concentrate on two particular aspects of the gait pattern, i.e. the angle and base of gait and the line of progression. First of all, in this instance, the leg and foot must be conceived as one unit whose position within the transverse body plane is governed by the torsional relationships of each segment along the length of the limb. These torsional relationships govern the angle at which the foot is placed on the ground. Therefore the foot can be abducted, adducted or straight in respect to the mid-line of the body (this is not taking into consideration supination or pronation within the foot itself). If this torsional relationship is not ideal, then the most functionally effective way to alter it is at the phase of gait when the limb becomes a propulsive lever, and the foot is required to flex at the metatarsophalangeal joints. So in this form of therapy we are looking at a way of changing the angle at which the foot is functioning as it travels from mid-stance into the propulsive phase of gait. In doing this, we can also subtly change and improve the position of heel-strike to a more conventional attitude as the same foot follows through after the swing phase. Furthermore, we are, at the point of propulsion, also controlling the point of optimum function of knee extension, which is otherwise put out of true extension timing by an abducted or adducted foot.

Following this concept, we can see that an incorrect transverse plane relationship of the foot and leg is sustained in the unshod foot; such unusual positions are managed functionally by the innate ability of the foot to attempt compensation for an abnormality above it. The foot shod in a flexible shoe is no more assisted in overcoming any of these anomalies than is the unshod foot. However, by governing the point at which the shoe flexes, it is possible to force the limb to twist inwards or outwards in which ever way is desired for correction. (The line along which the shoe flexes is termed, the 'break-line'.) We can examine this diagramatically (Fig. 11.7).

There are two ways in which the angle of shoe flexion, the 'break-line', can be controlled:

a. By stiffening the sole of the shoe to prevent flexion along any line other than that in which it is desired to produce correction.
b. By the use of an orthosis with a suitably angled anterior border. This orthosis achieves the desired result by acting as a rigid shank, or stiffener, for the sole of the shoe.

The first option of stiffening the sole of the shoe is satisfactory, but limits the therapeutic action to the pair of shoes on which the modifi-

▨ Stiffening applied to sole

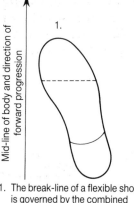 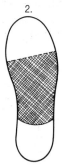 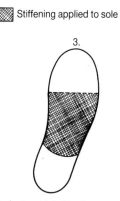

Mid-line of body and direction of forward progression

1. The break-line of a flexible shoe is governed by the combined influence of the transverse plane relationship of the foot to the ground and the direction of forward progression of the body

2. The break-line can be chosen and the sole proximal to it stiffened to prevent flexion from occurring anywhere else

3. The foot restricted by the predetermined break-line must twist outwards to allow flexion to occur. As the foot moves into the propulsive phase of gait this will improve its relationship to the forward line of progression of the body

Fig. 11.7 In-toeing gait.

cation has been performed. The more versatile option is to produce an orthosis which can be moved from shoe to shoe and thus maintain the therapy, regardless of the footwear being worn.

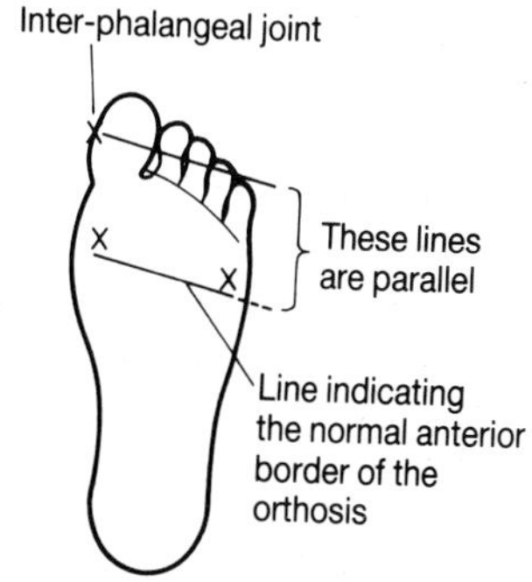

Casting technique and method of manufacture of the orthosis

The negative casts are taken in the semi-weight-bearing position with the foot positioned in biomechanical normality. This has already been described. Once the positive cast has set, any surface discrepancies must be made good. The cast must then be modified slightly, but before any plaster is added two lines must be drawn on the plantar surface of the cast, one line in the position of the normal anterior border of an orthosis, and another line which is parallel to this one but begins at the interphalangeal joint of the first toe and runs across to the fifth toe. This line must be drawn now so that if the fifth toe is short it will be noticed, as the line will run distal to it (Fig. 11.8). A short toe will cause difficulties in the manufacture of the device.

The cast must now be modified in the area between the plantar surface of the metatarsophalangeal joints and the plantar surface of the apex of the toes. The natural depression in this area must be filled with plaster of Paris to render it flat. If this is not done, the shell material will sink into the depression when being 'pressed' and cause discomfort to the wearer. Also at this time, the length of the fifth toe must be extended, if it is short, so that it reaches just distal to the line drawn across from the first toe. However, it should not be increased in width at all (Fig. 11.9).

Once the modification is finished and has been smoothed, the lines drawn before the modification was performed should be redrawn, or reinforced, and marks made on the more distal line which correspond to the most medial side of the interphalangeal joint on the first toe and, on the lateral side, the widest point of the fifth toe. The marking-out procedure now differs, depending on whether you are treating an in-toeing or out-toeing gait anomaly.

Inter-phalangeal joint

These lines are parallel

Line indicating the normal anterior border of the orthosis

Fig. 11.8

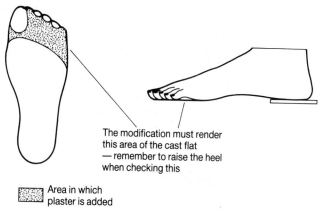

The modification must render this area of the cast flat — remember to raise the heel when checking this

Area in which plaster is added

Fig. 11.9 Modification of the cast.

In-toeing (more common)

A line is drawn from the point indicating the normal medial anterior border of an orthosis, diagonally across to the mark made on the distal lateral side of the fifth toe. A ruler should be used. With the ruler in position, a diagonal line may then be drawn (Fig. 11.10).

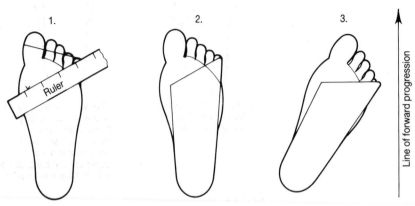

1. The re-defined anterior border of the orthosis is marked with the help of a ruler

2. The remaining marking-out is done normally except for the lateral side which is widened to correspond to the width of the lateral side of the anterior border

3. The foot must now twist outwards to re-establish the flexion line at its correct relationship to the line of forward progression

Fig. 11.10

This diagonal line represents the anterior border of the orthosis, and because the orthosis is made from a rigid material it will cause the foot to abduct in order to achieve flexion at the point of propulsion. The remaining marking out of the cast is done normally, except for the lateral side, which is widened to correspond to the width of the redefined lateral anterior border of the orthosis. The shell is then pressed and machined, particular care being taken to produce a smooth, sympathetic 'top' bevel to the anterior border.

(The angle of the anterior border may be altered as desired, to achieve the required amount of correction.)

Out-toeing

It is rare for this gait abnormality to require treatment. However, when out-toeing is excessive, then assistance can be given to bring the feet back to a less abducted position.

The orthosis is 'marked-out' as follows:

A line is drawn from the point indicating the lateral anterior border of a normal orthosis, diagonally across to the mark made on the medial side of the interphalangeal joint on the first toe (Fig. 11.11).

The diagonal line represents the anterior border of the orthosis and will cause a reduction in abduction of the foot in order to achieve

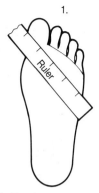
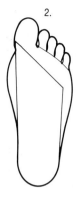
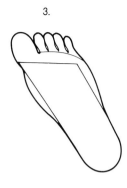

1. The re-defined anterior border is marked with the help of a ruler

2. The remaining marking-out is done normally except for the medial side of the orthosis which may need to be widened to correspond with the medial side of the anterior border

3. The foot must now twist inwards to achieve a flexion line which is nearer to the correct relationship with the natural line of progression

Fig. 11.11

flexion at the point of propulsion. The foot will not be adducted with respect to the mid-line of the body (as shown in the intentionally exaggerated diagram), but brought into a less abducted position. The angle of the anterior border can be adjusted on fitting, to achieve the desired correction. It is prudent to over-correct initially, to re-educate the phyasic activity of the musculature. The remaining marking-out is done normally, except that the medial side of the orthosis is widened to meet the medial edge of the anterior border.

The shell may then be pressed and machined.

SUMMARY

The aim of this type of orthosis as a means of repositioning the foot at the point of propulsion can be a useful means of assisting in the treatment of these gait abnormalities. I should point out that, when treating in-toeing gait, thought should be given to the design of the orthosis, to prevent the tendency the child will have to pronate excessively once the improved transverse plane position has been established. If considered necessary, the shell shape described for the hypermobile foot should be used, with the anterior border modified as just described. Examination of the ranges of motion of the relevant joints, and careful examination of the range of dorsiflexion at the ankle, will aid in the design.

In this chapter the shell shapes required for different therapeutic needs have been discussed. For you, I am sure, this is just the beginning; because once you have caught the excitment posed by the range of possibilities, and grasped the mechanical diversity of your medium, then experimentation will lead you as far as you wish to travel.

What is discussed in this chapter is the range of therapeutic possibilities you have at your disposal when working in the field of biomechanics. While your medium is the foot, it is impossible to divorce yourself from the effect your therapy will be having on the mechanics of the lower limb as a whole; neither is it desirable. The optimum functional position of the foot, once restored, may achieve improved function and relief of symptoms elsewhere in the limb. Indeed, such means of therapy can be used with this direct therapeutic aim. Furthermore, once the mechanics of the limb have been mastered, the optimum functional position of the foot can sometimes be traded to achieve a therapeutic advantage in the joints associated with gait elsewhere along the length of the limb.

12

The issuing and 'wearing-in' of orthoses

It can take some time for patients to become used to wearing functional foot orthoses. Just as the eyes must adapt to the wearing of spectacles which transform the way the viewer perceives the environment, so too must the limbs adapt to a new way in which they react to their own environment, the ground. Be it a matter of 'fine' tuning the mechanics of the limbs or compromising for an irreparable structural or mechanical fault in this mechanism of levers, the change can seldom be brought about instantaneously. Time must be allowed for the patient to adapt to the altered range of motion, and to blend the individual segments into a new and more efficient and harmonious interaction. It is vital that both you and your patients understand this.

The subsequent pages contain ideas which are based on experience, which may help you to guide your patients into the successful use of these devices.

RIGID AND SEMI-FLEXIBLE ORTHOSES

In most cases the orthoses should be worn for one hour only on the first day of issue. This is then increased by one hour each day, so that on the day after issue the patient is wearing the orthoses for two hours, and so on. This hour per day increase is continued until the orthoses are being worn comfortably all day.

Sometimes, because a relatively large degree of correction is being attempted, the patient may find that wearing the orthoses for this long each day and increasing the length of time worn at the rate mentioned is too sudden a change to be comfortable. The symptoms can vary, but may manifest themselves as aching in the knees (common), hips, thighs and back after three to four consecutive hours of wear. Discomfort may also be felt on the plantar surface of the foot. Therefore, depending on the type and severity of the symptoms demonstrated, a compromise must be sought, to allow a comfortable wearing-in period.

If the symptoms are only mild, my advice is not to increase the length of time worn from three hours for at least two days. When the orthoses are being worn for three hours with comfort, I then ask my patients to increase the time by three-quarters of an hour daily, instead of an hour. Furthermore, during the 'wearing in' exercise, I like all patients to wear the orthoses for half an hour in the evening while relaxing, in order to maintain the development of the structural realignment being attempted. If symptoms are severe, I advise halving the time being worn, and holding at that level until worn with comfort. (For instance, if three hours of wear causes severe discomfort, then the time will be reduced to one and a half hours until the orthoses are worn with comfort for this reduced time.) This is then increased by half an hour per day. Normally, I like, and feel it is therapeutically wise, to pre-empt the situations when the wearing-in time should be more gradual. This also develops the patient's confidence. In more marked deformities it can be prudent to prescribe daily increase times of half an hour right from the start. This prevents discomfort and subsequent 'back-tracking' or, worse still, rejection by the patient of a device which will ultimately be of benefit to them.

In my opinion, when treating children and handicapped people (both mentally and physically) it is essential that a responsible parent or guardian is informed of the 'wearing-in' requirements, so as to assist in the process. The time spent in discussion, explanation and counselling is as essential as the painstaking prescription and manufacture of these devices. In these situations it is wise to restrict the wearing of the orthoses to *home only* until five consecutive hours of wear have been achieved with comfort. This allows more careful monitoring by the parent or guardian.

In all cases, I like to see my patients within a month of the issue of their orthoses. At this time, progress can be checked and any small problems solved. I always instil in my patients a relaxed attitude towards my willingness to talk with them by telephone about their treatment during this period of adjustment. The more demanding cases I normally contact myself after the first week of issue, to enquire as to their progress. This, I find, helps to alleviate any small but potentially troublesome problems they may be experiencing, some of which they feel are too small to bother me with.

From time to time, particularly while you are gaining clinical experience, it may be necessary to make slight adjustments to the posting angulations of the orthoses. However, do not be hasty in making any alterations. If all the diagnostic and therapeutic criteria have been met, and the manufacture has been painstaking, it is possible with careful management to guide your patients through the initial period. Belief in oneself is paramount, and this will be forthcoming if biomechanical principles are clearly understood and the measurement details mentioned in the text are accurate. Clear and thorough diagnosis in any medical treatment is paramount. If you have been conscientious, trust your judgement. However, if after six to eight weeks the orthoses persist in causing discomfort, you would be wise to re-examine your patient and, if necessary, make adjustments to the orthoses or remake them.

ACCOMMODATIVE ORTHOSES

Accommodative orthoses do not generally require such a gradual adjustment programme as do rigid and semi-flexible orthoses.

These appliances are usually prescribed in order to accommodate an existing deformity (when no range of motion is available to allow improvement), to provide shock absorbtion or to redistribute pressure away from prominent lesions. As the materials are softer, the unyielding biomechanical control of the rigid and semi-flexible orthosis is not present, and the foot is able to adapt more easily to the device.

Therefore, when issuing orthoses of this type, I normally allow my patients to wear them all day right from the first day of issue. However, if some significant mechanical control has been incorporated into the device, I follow the 'wearing-in' programme already described for rigid and semi-flexible orthoses.

THE WEARING OF ORTHOSES FOR SPORT

Many sports shoes have inside them an inner-sole made out of a soft thermoplastic material. When functional orthoses are to be used in sports shoes, it is important to remove this inner-sole before inserting the orthosis. This not only prevents crowding of the foot in the shoe, but maintains the efficient functioning of the posts, which if placed on top of a soft inner-sole will sink into it in stance, thus reducing the therapeutic value of the orthosis.

It is important to explain to your patients the difference between everyday use and wearing the orthoses for their sporting activity. Firstly, the wearing-in should have reached the point where the orthoses are being worn comfortably for a full day before sporting use is attempted. The increased stress the limbs are subjected to in sport may precipitate some adjustment problems if the orthoses are used too early, before the limbs have had time to adapt to their improved functioning position. Importantly, the foot which acts as the medium by which the angular change to the limb is achieved may experience blistering from the redirection of the forces acting upon it.

I would suggest therefore that, after the orthoses have been worn comfortably for at least eight hours, they are inserted in the sports shoes for one quarter of the time spent in participation in sport. This means that if the sporting activity lasts for one hour, the orthoses are worn for quarter of an hour; or, if easier, say the distance run is 4 kilometres, the orthoses are worn for 1 kilometre. The duration of wear is then increased by a further one quarter every three days, if, and only if, the patient is comfortable at the 'wearing' time reached at that point. Done in this way, approximately two weeks will elapse before the orthoses are being worn for the duration of the sporting activity (assuming that the activity is pursued daily).

SUMMARY

Overall, your patients will benefit from your guidance during the early period of wear, and if and when adjustments are made to the orthoses, owing to improved function of the limbs, they will be confident and knowledgeable in the method of adaptation.

13
Common problems

Throughout the foregoing text I have stressed that the use of functional foot orthoses as a means of therapy is based on scientific and mechanical principles. The practitioner who becomes adept in the design, prescription and manufacture of these devices will achieve therapeutic success and much personal enjoyment. However, there will be times, particularly when beginning, when problems arise with the orthoses after they have been issued and worn. The more common of these problems are listed below, together with their causes and their remedies.

Problem	Cause	Remedy
1. Shell material fractures	a. Choice of shell material is inappropriate b. Pronation allowance is inadequate	a. Reassess choice, relating it to the weight-to-thickness ratio b. Check the pronatory rock of the orthosis; if this is adequate, the reason will lie in the shell material
2. Anterior border of the shell of the orthosis 'cuts into' the skin just proximal to the metatarsal heads	a. Shell of the orthosis is too short. b. The fore-foot posting is sufficiently high to require a fore-foot extension and this has not been added. c. Top bevel on the anterior border is too abrupt	a. Examine the length and flexibility of the foot; there may be elongation occurring on weight bearing. Remake if too short b. Apply fore-foot extension, if required, for sympathetic blending of fore-foot post c. Re-machine the top bevel to produce a more gentle blending
3. Anterior border of the orthosis digs into the plantar surface of the metatarsal heads when standing	Shell of the orthosis is too long	Adjust to the correct dimensions
4. Pressure or a pinching sensation is felt around the heel seat of the orthosis	Heel seat of the orthosis is too narrow because insufficient tissue spread was allowed around the heel when the positive cast was modified	Re-modify the heel area of the positive cast, and remake the orthosis

5. Heel rides out of the shoe when walking

a. Heel area of the orthosis and/or rear-foot post is too thick
b. Excessive convex curvature of the plantar surface of the heel of the orthosis is present. This occurs sometimes when the negative cast is taken in a non-weight-bearing position
c. Too much plaster has been added around the perimeter of the heel during the positive cast modification. This has made the heel of the orthosis too wide, preventing it from sitting correctly in the heel seat of the shoe
d. Height of the heel counter of the shoe is too low to allow the use of orthoses. This can happen with some fashion shoes

a. If possible, reduce the thickness
b. Grind away some of the curvature in the method described for intrinsically posting the rear-foot. Then remake the orthosis.

c. Remove the excess plaster of Paris and remake the orthosis

d. Give advice on more suitable footwear

6. Orthosis squeaks in the shoe when the patient is walking

Movement of the orthosis in the shoe causes rubbing on the upper material

Apply some talcum powder to the edge of the orthosis, or rub a bar of soap around the edge of the orthosis before replacing the device in the footwear

7. Patient has the sensation that the foot is sliding off the lateral side of the orthosis

Excessive pronation is occurring in a hypermobile foot, or there is present a structural abduction of the fore-foot

Remake the orthosis and incorporate a high lateral flange as described in the section on 'unusual shell shapes'

8. Foot slides forward on the orthosis during gait

a. Slip-on style of footwear is being worn
b. Orthosis is slippery

c. Apex of the convex curve of the plantar surface of the heel of the orthosis is positioned too distally.

Cross section of shell

Ground

Apex of curve too distal   Slope created

This creates a slope on which the patient's heel slides down during gait
d. height of the heel of the shoe is excessive

a. Advise the patient to wear shoes with fastenings.
b. Apply a 'top-split' grain leather top cover.
c. Examine the positive cast and, if necessary, reshape this area to position the apex of this curve in the centre of the heel seat. Remake the orthosis

Ground

Apex of curve positioned centrally

d. Encourage your patient to obtain shoes with a heel height not in excess of 30 mm

9. Orthosis slips forward in the shoe

a. Incorrect sagittal angulation of the inferior surface of the heel post for the height of the heel of the shoe
b. Rear-foot of the orthosis is posted intrinsically and the shell material has a low coefficient of friction

a. Apply a new heel post and re-machine

b. Roughen the inferior surface of the heel of the shell by grinding on an abrasive wheel, or stick a piece of sand-screen abrasive cloth to the inferior surface of the heel

10. Pain is felt under the shaft of the first metatarsal

a. Rigid plantar-flexed first ray has not been taken into account when manufacturing the shell
b. Insufficient cast modification has been performed in this area
c. Wearing-in time of orthosis too short
d. Posting of the fore-foot is too severe or incorrect

e. A pronation allowance has not been made at the fore-foot post
f. The curve created by the intrinsic fore-foot post is too abrupt
g. The orthosis is too wide and is being 'held' by the upper of the shoe

a. Remove the shell material in the manner described in the section on 'unusual shell shapes'
b. Re-modify the cast and remake the orthosis
c. Follow the wearing-in instructions
d. Check the measurements and ranges of motion of the joints associated with gait. Adjust the posting, if necessary
e. Machine this allowance in the proper way
f. Re-modify the cast and re-make the orthosis

g. Check the width, and reduce if necessary

11. Pain is felt in the whole of the medial longitudinal arch

a. Poor cast modification and insufficient plaster added in the arch
b. A flexible cavus foot

c. An equinus foot type in which the plantar fascia becomes very prominent when the foot is bearing weight

a. Re-modify and remake the orthosis

b. Modify the cast by adding slightly more plaster in the medial arch to allow for the elongation of the foot on weight bearing
c. Dorsiflex the foot to resistance and then dorsiflex the toes. Measure the distance the plantar fascia rises from the plantar surface of the foot and modify the cast accordingly. Make the orthosis from EVA with a softer density of material in the mid-foot. Negative cast can be taken in a semi-weight-bearing position if required. Still make the orthosis out of EVA

12. Wear plate cracks or the hard plugs placed on the medial side of the rear-foot post, to resist pronation, break through the wear plate

This is inevitable after 12 months of continuous wear

Replace the wear plate

(continued on p. 172)

13. Foot sits too far forward on the heel seat of the orthosis, leaving a gap between the heel of the patient and the back of the shoe

a. This is commonly seen when using EVA, if the perimeter of the heel seat of the orthosis is left too wide

Width too great

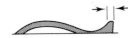

Sagittal section through orthosis

b. Tapering around the edge of the heel post does not match the shape of the heel seat of the shoe

Cross section through edge of

heel seat

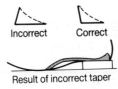

Incorrect   Correct

Result of incorrect taper

c. Poor cast modification

a. Reduce the width until the correct fit is achieved

b. Taper it correctly to fit the shoe

c. Examine the positive cast and re-modify it if necessary

14. Dorsum of the toes becomes rubbed on the upper of the shoe

Fore-foot posting is too severe, reducing the depth of the shoe and allowing insufficient room for the toes, and/or the toe-box of the shoe is too shallow to accommodate orthoses

Adjust the posting accordingly, or acquire a deeper shoe if the posting cannot be compromised

15. Pain is felt in the metatarsophalangeal joint of the first toe

A significant varus fore-foot post has been applied without a fore-foot extension and due consideration being given to the function of the first toe; this may be causing hallux flexus

Extend the fore-foot post to the end of the first toe, or all the toes, depending on the clinical findings

Further reading

Albert S 1981 A subjective comparison of Spenco and P P T soft tissue supplements used in footgear. Orthotics and Prosthetics 35(3): 17–21

Anderson H et al 1976 An introduction to medical sciences for clinical practice—the musculoskeletal system. Year Book Medical Publishers, Chicago

Ansin K M 1983 The origin of the concept of the neutral sub-talar joint position. Footprint 1(1): 9–26

Asher C 1975 Postural variations in childhood. Butterworth, London

Barham J N 1978 Mechanical kinesiology. C.V. Mosby, St Louis

Black J, Dumbleton J H 1981 Clinical biomechanics. Churchill Livingstone, Edinburgh

Black J A 1987 The influence of the sub-talar joint on running injuries of the lower limb. Chiropodist 42(2): 43–48

Blakeman P D 1985 Forces, stress and appliance materials. Chiropodist 40(5): 132–136

Boyce N R 1986 Efficient orthoses—biomechanics in practice. Chiropodist 41(10): 385–388

Bradley M A, Bader D L 1986 The measurement of foot pressures. Chiropodist 41(9): 335–346

Brand P W 1966 Insensitive feet. The leprosy mission.

Broer M R 1969 Efficiency of human movement. W B Saunders, Philadelphia

Cailliett R 1968 Foot and ankle pain. F A Davis, Philadelphia

Cailliett R 1973 Knee pain and disability. F A Davis, Philadelphia

Campbell G et al 1982 Compression testing of foamed plastics and rubbers for use as orthotic insoles. Prosthetics and Orthotics International 6: 48–52

Carlson S 1972 How man moves. Heinemann, London

Carrel J M 1978 Questions and answers in podiatric orthopedics. Futura, Mt Kisco, New York

Ceeney E 1958 An introduction to shoe fitting. Pitman, London

Cochran G V B 1982 A primer of orthopaedic biomechanics. Churchill Livingstone, Edinburgh

Copeman W S C 1970 Textbook of the rheumatic diseases. E & S Livingstone, Edinburgh

Crawford Adams J 1971 Outline of orthopaedics. Churchill Livingstone, Edinburgh

Daniels L, Worthington C 1980 Muscle testing, 4th edn. W B Saunders, Philadelphia

Dick W C 1972 An introduction to clinical rheumatology. Churchill Livingstone, Edinburgh

Dickson J 1974 Proprioceptive control of human movement. Lupus Books, London

Ducroquet R et al 1968 Walking and limping. J B Lippincott, Philadelphia

Faris I 1982 The management of the diabetic foot. Churchill Livingstone, Edinburgh

Frederick E C 1984 Sports shoes and playing surfaces. Human Kinetics, Champaign, Illinois

Fritschi E P 1971 Reconstructive surgery in leprosy. Wright, Bristol

Gamble F O, Yale I 1978 Clinical foot roentgenology. Williams and Wilkins, Baltimore

Gowitzke B A, Milner M 1980 Understanding the scientific bases of human movement, 2nd edn. Williams and Wilkins, Baltimore

Hamilton W C 1984 Traumatic disorders of the ankle. Springer-Verlag, New York

Hamner C et al 1987 Appliance materials research project. Chiropodist 42(2): 51–54

Hawkins C, Currey H L F 1971 Reports on rheumatic diseases. The Arthritis and Rheumatic Council for Research, London

Helfet A J, Gruebel Lee D H 1980 Disorders of the foot. J B Lipincott, Philadelphia

Higgins J R 1977 Human movement. C V Mosby, St Louis

Hlavac H F 1977 The foot book. World Publications, Mountain View, California

Hoppenfeld S 1976 Physical examination of the spine and extremities. Appleton-Century-Croft, New York

Inman V T 1976 The joints of the ankle. Williams and Wilkins, Baltimore

Inman V T, et al 1981 Human walking. Williams and Wilkins, Baltimore

Julian C M 1987 The wearing of neutral talus orthoses. Reprint series. The New Zealand School of Podiatry

Kapandji I A 1970 The physiology of the joints. Vol 3: The trunk and vertebral column. Churchill Livingstone, Edinburgh

Le Bendig M, Diamond E 1976 A podiatric resource guide for preventive and rehabilitative foot and leg care. Futura, Mt Kisco, New York

Lehmkuhl L D, Smith L K 1984 Brunnstrom's clinical kinesiology, 4th edn. F A Davis, Philadelphia

Lloyd-Roberts G C, Ratcliff A H C 1978 Hip disorders in children. Butterworth, London

McMinn R M H et al 1982 A colour atlas of foot and ankle anatomy. Wolfe Medical, London

McRae R 1976 Clinical orthopaedic examination. Churchill Livingstone, Edinburgh

Medical Research Council 1974 Aids to the investigation of peripheral nerve injuries. Her Majesty's Stationery Office, London

Minns R J et al 1986 A study of foot shape, underfoot pressure patterns, lower limb rotations and gait in children. Chiropodist 41(3): 89–99

Mitchell B 1970 Today's athlete. Pelham Books, London

Munzenberg K J 1985 The orthopaedic shoe. VCH Publishers

Napier J 1967 The antiquity of human walking. Scientific American Offprints. W H Freeman, San Francisco

Neale D 1985 Common foot disorders. Churchill Livingstone, Edinburgh

Nigg B M 1986 Biomechanics of running shoes. Human Kinetics, Champaign, Illinois

Payne C B 1982 Biomechanics of the foot and related pathology. Podiatry Associates, Riccarton, New Zealand

Piasaniello D L, Van Essen A 1987 Possible health risks associated with techniques employed in the fabrication of podiatric orthotic devices. Australian Podiatrist 21(1): 10–19

Rakow R 1979 Podiatric management of the diabetic foot. Futura, New York

Redford J B 1980 Orthotics etcetera. Williams and Wilkins, Baltimore

Robbins J H 1983 Clinical handbook of podiatric medicine. Ohio College of Podiatric Medicine

Root M C et al 1977 Clinical biomechanics. Vol 2: Clinical Biomechanics Corporation, California

Root M C et al 1971 Neutral position casting techniques. Clinical Biomechanics Corporation

Rose G K 1986 Orthotics (principles and practice). Heinemann, London

Rowe K 1987 Peroneal spastic flat-foot. Chiropodist 42(1): 15–19

Sgarlato T E 1971 Compendium of podiatric biomechanics. California College of Podiatric Medicine

Sheenan G 1972 The encyclopaedia of athletic medicine. Anderson World Inc.

Sinclair D 1973 Human growth after birth. Oxford University Press, Oxford

Simkin A, Stokes I A F 1981 The dynamic force distribution level when walking under normal and rheumatic feet. Rheumatology and Rehabilitation 20: 88–97

Subotnick S I 1979 Cures for common running injuries. Anderson World Inc.

Subotnick S I 1977 The running foot doctor. World Publications, Mountain View, California

Sutherland D H 1984 Gait disorders in childhood and adolescence. Williams and Wilkins, Baltimore

Tax H R 1980 Podopediatrics. Williams and Wilkins, Baltimore

Thompson C W 1985 Manual of structural kinesiology, 10th edn. Times Mirror/Mosby College Publishing

Tillman K 1979 The rheumatoid foot. Georg Thieme, Stuttgart

Turco V J 1981 Clubfoot. Churchill Livingstone, Edinburgh

United States manufacturing company Technical manual for vacuum forming of plastics in orthotics and prosthetics

Warwick R, Williams P L 1973 Gray's anatomy, 35th edition. Longman, London

Watkins J 1983 An introduction to mechanics of human movement. MTP Press, Lancaster

Weed J H et al 1978 A biplanar grind for
rear posts on a functional orthosis.
Journal of the American Podiatry
Association 69(1): 35–39

Wheeler J R 1984 The New Zealand road
to fitness. Stortford Publications

Weissman S D 1983 Radiology of the
foot. Williams and Wilkins, Baltimore

Whitney A K 1979 Biomechanical
footwear balancing. Pennsylvania
College of Podiatric Medicine

Yablon I G et al 1983 Ankle injuries.
Churchill Livingstone, Edinburgh

Yale I, Yale J F 1984 The arthritic foot.
Williams and Wilkins, Baltimore

Index